THE
ENZYME
FACTOR

THE ENZYME FACTOR

Hiromi Shinya, MD

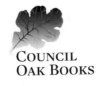

COUNCIL
OAK BOOKS

SAN FRANCISCO & TULSA

Council Oak Books, LLC
www.counciloakbooks.com

©2005, 2007, 2010 by Hiromi Shinya
Portions originally published in Japanese by Sunmark Press
First paperback edition, third printing 2011

Designed by Carl Brune

Printed in Canada

ISBN 978-0-9822900-3-3

LIBRARY OF CONGRESS CATALOGING-IN-PUBLICATION DATA
Shinya, Hiromi.
  [Byoki ni naranai ikikata. English]
  The enzyme factor / Hiromi Shinya. -- 1st English-language ed.
    p. cm.
  "Originally published in Japanese by Sunmark Press."
  ISBN-13: 978-1-57178-209-0 (hardcover : alk. paper)
  ISBN-10: 1-57178-209-5
  1. Enzymes--Popular works. 2. Health--Popular works.
3. Nutrition--Popular works. I. Title.
  QP601.S4764 2005
  612.0151--dc22
    2007015949

Notice: This book is intended as a reference volume only, not as a medical manual. The information presented here is designed to help you make informed decisions about your health. It is not intended as a substitute for any treatment that may have been prescribed by your doctor, who is acquainted with your specific needs. If you suspect that you have a medical problem, we urge you to seek competent medical care.

Contents

Publisher's Note

To gastroenterologists and surgeons worldwide, Hiromi Shinya, M.D. needs no introduction. As the pioneer of colonoscopic surgery (he developed the technique —which, in fact, is named for him — and helped design the instrument used), he is widely acknowledged to be one of the world's leading physicians.

Dr. Shinya has been in the regular practice of medicine for over four decades, treating presidents, prime ministers, movie stars, musicians, and many, many less well-known patients. In fact, he has examined the stomachs and intestines of over 300,000 people. Currently, he is Clinical Professor of Surgery at Albert Einstein College of Medicine in New York City and Chief of the Surgical Endoscopy Unit at Beth Israel Medical Center.

Through vast experience with hundreds of thousands of patients, some of whom he has followed over a lifetime, Dr. Shinya has developed and tested clinically an approach to health based on the body's supply of a vital enzyme, which he has termed the "miracle" enzyme. This enzyme, he believes, is the key to a long and healthy life.

His purpose in writing *The Enzyme Factor* is to explain the workings of this enzyme and why it is so important to human health. He sees this publication as the culmination of his life's work, extending his discoveries to millions of people whom he will never be able to treat personally. In this book, Dr. Shinya details a lifestyle that can ensure better health and explains why these practices are so powerful.

Born in Japan and practicing medicine half of each year in Tokyo, Dr. Shinya brings the perspectives of both Eastern and Western medicine to his work on human health. He first wrote this book in Japanese. The Japanese version has been a sensation, selling over two million copies within months of its publication. Council Oak is honored to be able to present *The Enzyme Factor* in English. Along with Hiromi Shinya, M.D., we hope that this book will guide you to your happy and healthy lifestyle.

Preface

I came of age in Japan just after the war, when American technologies and customs were transforming my native land. I wanted to study medicine in America. I took a medical degree in Japan, then, in 1963, moved to the United States with my young bride to start the surgical residency program at the Beth Israel Medical Center in New York.

Coming to the U.S. from a foreign country, I understood that I had to try hard and be really good to be respected as a surgeon in America. Growing up I had studied martial arts and, because of that training, I learned to use each hand equally well. Being ambidextrous enabled me to perform surgery with unusual efficiency.

During my residency, I assisted Dr. Leon Ginsburg, one of the discoverers (with Drs. Burrill Bernard Crohn and Gordon Oppenheimer) of Crohn's disease. One day the chief resident and the senior resident who usually assisted Dr. Ginsburg couldn't assist in the operating room, so Dr. Ginsburg's nurse, who had seen me work, recommended me. Being ambidextrous, I finished very quickly. At first Dr. Ginsburg couldn't believe it was done correctly in such a short operation and he was angry, but when he saw how well the patient healed without the excessive bleeding and swelling that follows a lengthy surgery, he was impressed. I started working with him regularly.

Neither my wife nor our baby daughter did well in the United States. My wife was sick much of the time, weak, and she couldn't breast feed, so we gave our daughter baby formula made from cow's milk. I would work all day at the hospital and come home and help my wife who was pregnant again. I changed the diapers and gave the baby a bottle, but my daughter cried a lot and then she developed a rash all over her skin. She was itching and miserable.

Then my son was born. His arrival was a joy, but before long he developed rectal bleeding. About that time I had acquired the first primitive colonoscope, so I was able to examine my little son and found an inflammation of the colon, or ulcerative colitis.

I was devastated. Here I was, a doctor, but I couldn't cure my beautiful young wife or relieve the suffering of my son or daughter. I hadn't learned anything in medical school that would tell me what was causing them to be sick. I consulted other doctors, the best I knew, but no one could help me. Being a skillful surgeon or giving medicine for symptoms was not enough. I wanted to know what caused disease.

In Japan I had never seen the kind of atrophic dermatitis that my daughter had, so I started investigating what in the U.S. could cause my daughter to have this. In Japan we didn't have much dairy food so I thought perhaps it was the cow's milk in her baby formula. When we took away the milk she quickly improved, and I realized she was allergic to the cow's milk. She couldn't digest it and undigested particles that were small enough to pass from her intestines into her blood were attacked by her immune system as if they were foreign invaders. The same thing turned out to be true with my son. When we stopped giving him milk his colitis disappeared.

My wife's illness was finally diagnosed as lupus. Her blood count would drop and she would become pale and anemic. She was in and out of the hospital as we struggled to save her life. She died before I knew enough to help her.

Even today I can't say what caused her lupus, but I do know that she was genetically predisposed to have an over-reactive immune system. She went to a Westernized convent school when she was growing up in Japan where they gave her lots of milk. No doubt she was allergic to milk, as her two children would later be. Exposed over and over again to a food that created an allergic reaction, her immune system must have been depleted, leaving her open to the autoimmune disease of lupus.

Because of these experiences, I began to understand how vital diet is to our health. That was over fifty years ago and in the years since, I have examined the stomachs and colons and taken the dietary history of more than 300,000 patients.

I've spent my life trying to understand the human body, health and disease. I started out focusing on disease — what caused it and how to cure it — but as I began to understand more fully how the body works as a whole system, I changed the way I treat disease. I saw that we medical professionals and our patients should spend more time understanding health than fighting disease.

We are born with the right to health; it is natural to be healthy. Once I started understanding health I began to be able to work with the body, helping it to rid itself of disease. Only the body can heal itself. As a doctor, I create a space for that healing to happen.

So I started out trying to understand disease, but eventually my research led me to what I believe is the key to health. This key is our body's own miracle enzyme.

We have over 5000 enzymes in the human body that create perhaps 25,000 different reactions. You could say that every action in our body is controlled by enzymes, but we know very little about them. I believe we create these different enzymes out of a base or source enzyme, which is more or less finite in our body. If we exhaust these source enzymes, they are not available in sufficient numbers to properly repair cells, so, over time, cancer and other degenerative diseases develop.

This, in a nutshell, is the enzyme factor.

When I help my colon cancer patients heal, I first remove the cancer from the colon, and then I put them on a very strict diet of high-enzyme, non-toxic food and water so that they have more source enzymes to use for repairing the body's cells. I do not believe in using strong drugs that defeat the immune system, because I see that the cancer in the colon did not happen as an accidental, isolated incident. The cancer in the colon is telling me the whole body's source enzyme supply is being depleted and can no longer repair the cells properly.

While I believe that we are born with a limited supply of this source enzyme and we should not deplete it with bad food, toxins, poor elimination and stress, I have come to understand something else. That something else is why I call this source enzyme a "miracle" enzyme. I have witnessed spontaneous healings and remissions of all kinds of disease. As I studied these healings further, I began to understand how such miracles can happen.

We have discovered DNA but we don't know really that much about it. There is much potential sleeping in our DNA that we don't yet understand. My research indicates that a surge of positive emotional energy, such as that arising from love, laughter, and joy, can stimulate our DNA to produce a cascade of our body's source enzyme — the miracle enzyme that acts as a bio-catalyst for repairing our cells. Joy and love can awaken a potential far beyond our current human understanding.

I will tell you in this book what to do every day, and what to eat, and what supplements and enzymes to take to support your miracle enzymes and your health. However, the most important thing I can tell you to live a long and healthy life is to do what makes you happy (even if that means you occasionally don't follow my other recommendations).

Play music. Make love. Have fun. Enjoy simple pleasures. Live life with passion. Remember that a happy and meaningful life is nature's way to human health. Joyful enthusiasm, rather than perfect adherence to some dietary regime, is the key to making the enzyme factor work for you.

DR. HIROMI SHINYA
June, 2007

Introduction

The Enzyme Factor — The Key to Life's Code

Your body has a miraculous ability to heal itself.

In fact, your body is the only healing system that can bring you back into balance when illness strikes. Medicine can support your body through an emergency, surgery can be necessary in certain circumstances, but it is only your own body that has the ability to heal.

I have seen this truth about healing over and over again in my practice of medicine. Approximately 35 years ago, I became the first person in the world to successfully excise a polyp using a colonoscope without having to perform an incision into the abdominal wall. At the time it was a very important event because I was able to remove the polyp without cutting open the abdomen, thus avoiding side effects that can come with open surgery. As the only physician with this skill at the time, I was suddenly in great demand. At the time, more than 10 million people in the U.S. alone needed colon examinations and many needed to have polyps removed. Patients started coming from everywhere for this less invasive procedure. Thus, still in my early thirties, I became the Chief of Surgical Endoscopy of Beth Israel Medical Center in New York, working at the hospital in the morning and at my private clinic in the afternoon, examining patients from morning until night. Over the course of decades in clinical practice, examining literally hundreds of thousands of people as a gastrointestinal endoscopist, I have learned that when a person's gastrointestinal system is clean, that person's body is easily able to fight off diseases of whatever type. On the other hand, when a person's gastrointestinal system is not clean, that person will be prone to suffer from some kind of disease.

To put it another way: A person with good gastrointestinal characteristics is mentally and physically healthy, but a person with bad characteristics is usually carrying some mental or physical problem. Conversely, a healthy person has good gastrointestinal characteristics

1

while those of an unhealthy person are bad. Obviously, then, maintaining good stomach and intestinal characteristics is directly related to maintaining one's overall health.

What, specifically, should a person do (or avoid doing) to maintain good stomach and intestinal characteristics? To learn answers, I have for years had my patients answer a questionnaire about their eating history and other aspects of lifestyle. Thanks to the results of these questionnaires, I have discovered a strong relationship between health and certain ways of eating and living.

What I am about to introduce in this book is my theory of how to live a long and healthy life, based on data I have gathered through my decades of medical practice. The data suggests that the entire body and its myriad functions can be understood using one key.

THAT KEY, THE KEY TO A LONG AND HEALTHY LIFE, CAN BE SUMMED UP IN ONE WORD: *ENZYMES*.

An *enzyme* is a generic term for a protein catalyst that is made within the cells of living things. Wherever there is life, whether in plants or animals, enzymes always exist. Enzymes take part in all actions necessary to maintain life, such as synthesis and decomposition, transportation, excretion, detoxification and supply of energy. Living things would not be able to sustain life without enzymes.

More than 5,000 kinds of these vital enzymes are created in the cells of our bodies, and we also produce enzymes using the ezymes in the foods that we consume daily. The reason there are so many types of enzymes is because each one has a special characteristic and unique function. For example, the digestive enzyme amylase, found in saliva, reacts only to carbohydrates. Fats and proteins are also digested by each of their own distinct enzymes.

Although it is believed that many kinds of enzymes are created in response to our bodies' needs, it is still not clear *how* they are created in the cells. I have a theory that might shed light on that process. I believe there is a source enzyme — an unspecialized prototype enzyme. Until this source enzyme is converted into a specific enzyme in response to a particular need, it has the potential to become *any* kind of enzyme.

My theory, developed through my years of clinical practice and observation, is this: Your health depends on how well you maintain—rather than exhaust—the source enzymes in your body. I use the term "source" enzymes for these catalysts, because they are, I believe, unspecialized enzymes that give rise to the more than 5,000 specialized enzymes that take on various activities within the human body. I also call them "miracle" enzymes, because they play a pivotal role in the body's ability to heal itself.

I first developed the idea of a source enzyme because I saw that when a particular area of the body is in need of and, therefore, consumes a large quantity of a specific type of enzyme, some other parts of the body tend to lack their own necessary enzymes. For example, if a large quantity of alcohol is consumed, a greater-than-normal amount of a particular enzyme is needed to break down the alcohol in the liver, creating a shortage of necessary enzymes for digestion and absorption in the stomach and intestines.

It seems that there is no set quantity of each of the several thousand kinds of enzymes in existence; rather, the source enzyme is converted into a particular type of enzyme when the need arises, and is consumed at the site where it is needed.

Currently, enzymes are attracting attention worldwide as the key element controlling our health, and although research continues to progress, there are many things we still do not understand about them. Dr. Edward Howell, a pioneer in enzyme research, proposed a truly interesting theory. It states that the number of enzymes a living thing can make during its lifetime is predetermined. Dr. Howell called this fixed number of body enzymes "enzyme potential." And when the enzyme potential is exhausted, that body's life ends.

Dr. Howell's theory is close to my theory of source enzymes, and, depending on which direction research goes, I anticipate that the existence of source enzymes will be proven. Although research on enzymes is still in its developmental stage, and the existence of the source enzyme is only a theory at present, nevertheless, abundant clinical evidence currently exists showing that we can tremendously strengthen our gastrointestinal characteristics — and thus our health — by following a diet that supplements enzymes, and mastering a lifestyle that does not exhaust the source enzyme.

The healthy lifestyle I discuss in this book consists of suggestions I have been making to my patients for years. I have seen many cures as a result of sick people adopting the practices I am about to suggest to you. Be prepared, however, to be surprised, as you may find some suggestions that seem to go against the prevailing wisdom regarding health and diet. I assure you that everything presented in this book has been verified. Only after verifying the safety of this lifestyle did I have my patients follow it — with remarkable results.

I myself follow this healthy lifestyle, and in the all the years I have practiced medicine, I have never even once been sick. The first and last time I received any medical treatment from a doctor was at the age of 19, when I had the flu. Now in my seventies, I still work in medical settings in both the U.S. and Japan. Although medicine is an extremely challenging profession, both physically and mentally, I have been able to maintain my health by daily practicing the good health lifestyle described in this book.

Having recognized via my own experience the lifestyle's positive effects, I have had my patients practice it as well. The results for my patients have been wonderful, far exceeding my own results. For example, having trained my patients to understand and follow this lifestyle, I have watched the cancer relapse rate among them fall to zero.

Although modern medicine is often practiced as if the body were a machine made up of independent parts, the human body is actually a single unit in which everything is linked together. For instance, the effects of an untreated cavity in just one tooth will spread throughout the entire body. Likewise, food that has been chewed insufficiently places a burden on the stomach and intestines, producing indigestion, blocking the absorption of vital nutrients, and resulting in myriad problems throughout the body. A small problem may seem irrelevant at first glance, but by no means is it rare for small problems to eventually lead to serious illnesses.

Our health is supported by various actions that occur ordinarily in our daily lives — eating, drinking, exercise, rest, sleep, and maintenance of a sound state of mind. If a problem develops in any one of these areas, it will affect the entire body. Given the complex interconnections within the human body, I believe that source enzymes carry out the function of maintaining the body's homeostasis — the balance necessary for a healthy life.

Unfortunately, modern society is overflowing with factors that consume our precious source enzymes. Alcohol, tobacco, drugs, food additives, agricultural chemicals, environmental pollution, electro-magnetic waves, and emotional stress are some of the factors that exhaust this enzyme. For you to maintain good health in contemporary society, it is essential to understand the mechanism of your own body and to exercise the will to look out for your own health.

Fortunately, this is not all that difficult to do. Once you clearly understand what exhausts source enzymes and how source enzymes can be supplemented, then, with just a little effort on a daily basis, you will be able to live out the rest of your natural life span *without getting sick*.

Our old saying needs updating: Instead of "eat, drink and be merry, for tomorrow you die," I suggest that you eat and drink wisely, and live merrily today and tomorrow. I would like to show you how to do just that.

Chapter 1

Enzymes and Your Health—
Misconceptions and Vital Truths

Forty years have passed since I became a gastrointestinal endoscopy specialist. In that time, I have worked closely with my patients to discover how to lead a healthy life. As a physician, I strongly believe that no matter how hard a doctor tries, he or she cannot maintain a patient's health over time just by doing checkups and treating diseases. Long-term health is the result of healthy attitudes and habits. Improving one's daily lifestyle is fundamentally more important than counting on the efficacy of surgery or medication.

The Enzyme Factor Diet and Lifestyle introduced in this book is able to report clinical results of a *0% cancer recurrence rate.*
I will say that again: *None* of my patients have had to face cancer again. Why? Because my cancer patients take their health condition seriously, place their full faith in supporting their body's healing, and practice my dietary health lifestyle daily. This is the healthy lifestyle I will teach you in this book, a simple set of new habits that will enable you to enjoy vital good health into very old age.

Armed with the knowledge in these pages, it will be up to you to choose sickness or health. In the past, people thought that illnesses could and should be cured solely by doctors and medication. Patients were passive, and simply took the doctor's instructions and the medication prescribed for them. However, we are now living in an era when all of us must take responsibility for our own health.

All of us hope we will never get sick—or, if we do, we have a strong desire to get better quickly. You may think this is impossible, but I assure you it is not. I propose in this book a way of life that will allow you to live out your natural life span without ever getting sick again.

Of course, in order to do this, it might be necessary to completely change the dietary habits and lifestyle you have pursued until now. Do not let the demands of this lifestyle cause you to consider forgoing my suggestions. Read on with an open mind. I firmly believe that by the time you finish reading this book, you will be inspired to make changes.

When people become sick, we often see them grieve over *why* they became sick. Being sick is not a test or punishment imposed by God. In most cases it is not preordained by genetics. Rather, almost all illness is the result of each person's habits that have accumulated over time.

You Can Become a Healthy 100-Year-Old

Do you consider yourself to be a healthy person? Not many people can answer this question with an unqualified "yes." Not many, I expect, because not being sick is not equivalent to being healthy. In Eastern medicine, there is a term "dormant illness." This term represents a condition in which a person is not yet sick and yet not completely healthy. In other words, it is a condition in which a person is but one step away from getting sick. Many Americans at present are actually in that condition.

Even people who consider themselves healthy are often troubled by such problems as chronic constipation or diarrhea, insomnia, and stiff necks and shoulders. These symptoms are SOS signals that your body is sending out. And if you make light of them by saying "this is normal for me" or "I'm usually like this," you run the risk of having the condition progress into a serious illness.

The average life expectancy in the United States rose dramatically, from 47 years in 1900 to almost 78 by 2006. Since it is in humankind's common interest for everyone to live longer, one could say this is a very positive trend.

However, the figures for average life expectancy should not make us complacent, because these numbers do not accurately reflect people's true health. For example, a 100-year-old person leading a healthy life and a 100-year-old who is sick and bedridden both count the same in life expectancy averages. Both are exactly the same age, but they do not have the same quality of life. If you are not healthy, you cannot make good use of the closing part of your long life. Very few people would want to live a long life if they were bedridden and suffering. Only when they are healthy do most people really want to live long lives.

Try to recall the appearance of an elderly relative or someone close to you. Looking at that person's health condition, would you be satisfied being in that same state when you reach their age? Unfortunately, most people would answer "no."

As one becomes older, even a healthy person's body will deteriorate. However, being sick and having your body experience a natural decline are two totally different things. My mother, who has followed this dietary lifestyle for many years, is healthy and active at age 96.

What causes elderly people to become sick?

The difference between a healthy centenarian and one who is bedridden is not a difference of age. It is a difference in eating and living habits that accumulate over that century. In short, whether a person is healthy or not depends on what that person eats and how that person lives day to day. What determines a person's state of health is the daily accumulation of things such as food, water, exercise, sleep, work, and stress.

If that is the case, then the question is what kind of lifestyle should we lead in order to live a long *and healthy* life?

Today's health and fitness industries have a huge market, with health products overflowing store counters. Many people buy health food supplements because labels tell them that a single remedy will address their health problems if they just drink or swallow that supplement each day. On top of that, when TV or magazine advertisements tell you that "xx product is good for your body," that product will often be sold out the next day. This means, in short, that most people do not really understand what is truly good for their bodies and are thus easily manipulated by the media.

WIDELY PROMOTED MISCONCEPTIONS ABOUT FOOD

Is there something you pay special attention to when trying to maintain your health? Are you conscientious about exercising regularly, eating properly and taking supplements and herbal medicine?

My intention is not to criticize your current dietary habits and lifestyle, but I highly recommend that at least once a day, you check your own health condition and contemplate whether your habits and lifestyle are truly effective in maintaining your health.

The reason I say this is that many products that are generally deemed "good for you" actually contain things that can damage your body.

COMMON MYTHS ABOUT FOOD

- Eat yogurt every day to improve digestion.

- Drink milk every day to avoid becoming calcium deficient.

- Get your daily vitamin through supplements rather than fruit, since fruit has a lot of carbohydrates and calories.

- Refrain from eating carbohydrates such as rice and bread in order to avoid gaining weight.

- Try to maintain a high protein diet.

- Get fluids from drinking Japanese green tea, which is rich in antioxidants.

- Boil tap water before drinking it to remove any chlorine remnants.

In fact, I have yet to meet a person who eats yogurt on a daily basis and still has good intestinal health. Many Americans have been drinking milk daily and eating dairy products since they were children, but many of these same people suffer from osteoporosis, which is supposed to be prevented by the calcium in milk. As a Japanese-American doctor, I treat patients in Tokyo during several months each year. I see that Japanese people who drink tea rich in antioxidants on a regular basis have very poor stomach characteristics as well. Tea instructors, for example, who drink large quantities of green tea as part of their work, often have what is known as atrophic gastritis, a precursor to stomach cancer.

Remember what over 300,000 clinical observations have told me: A person with poor gastrointestinal function is never healthy.

In light of this, why are things that damage your stomach and intestines widely considered to be good for your health? It is largely because people tend to look at only one aspect, or one effect, of that particular food or drink, rather than at the whole picture.

Take green tea as an example. There is no doubt that green tea, which contains many antioxidants, can kill bacteria and have positive anti-oxidation effects. As a result, there is a widespread belief that drinking a lot of Japanese green tea will prolong your life and may help prevent cancer. However, I have long had my doubts about this "antioxidant myth." Indeed, my own clinical data disprove this common belief. Through examining patients I have discovered that people who drink a lot of green tea have stomach problems.

It is true that antioxidants found in the tea are a type of polyphenol, which prevents or neutralizes the damaging effect of free radicals. However, when several of those antioxidants come together, they become something called tannin.

Tannin causes certain plants and fruits to have an astringent flavor. The "bitterness" of bitter persimmons, for example, is caused by tannin. Tannin is easily oxidized, so, depending on how much it is exposed to hot water or air, it can easily turn into tannic acid. Moreover, Tannic acid functions to coagulate proteins. My theory is that tea containing tannic acid has a negative effect on the gastric mucosa — the mucus membranes lining the stomach — causing the person to have stomach problems, such as ulcers.

The fact is, when I use an endoscope to examine the stomachs of people who regularly drink tea (green tea, Chinese tea, English black tea) or coffee containing lots of tannic acid, I usually find their gastric mucosa has thinned due to atrophic changes. That all-important stomach lining is literally wasting away. It is a well-known fact that chronic atrophic changes or chronic gastritis can easily become stomach cancer.

I am not the only medical professional to have noticed the ill effects of drinking coffee and tea. At the Japanese Cancer Conference in September 2003, Professor Masayuki Kawanishi of Mie University's School of Hygiene presented a report stating that *antioxidants can damage DNA*. Moreover, many kinds of teas that are sold in the supermarket today use agricultural chemicals during the cultivation process.

When you consider the effects of tannic acid, agricultural chemical remnants and caffeine put together, you know why I strongly recommend drinking plain water instead of tea. However, for those of you who like tea and cannot stop drinking it, I advise you to use organically grown tea leaves, drink it after meals instead of on an empty stomach to avoid excess stress on your stomach lining, and limit it to about 2-3 cups per day.

Many people fall for mistaken common beliefs regarding their health because medicine today does not look at the human body as a whole. For many years there has been a trend for doctors to specialize, looking at and treating just one part of the body. We can't see the forest for the trees. Everything in the human body is interconnected. Just because a component found in a food helps one part of the body function well, it does not mean that it is good for the entire body. When picking your food and drink, consider the big picture. You cannot decide whether a food is good or bad simply by looking at one ingredient found in that food.

EATING MEAT WILL NOT GIVE YOU STAMINA

In 1977, a very interesting report about food and health was published in America — the McGovern Report.

This report was published because a problem was brewing in the U.S. America's medical costs were putting enormous pressure on the economy. Despite medical advancements, the number of people getting sick, especially with cancer and heart disease, continued to increase every year. It was clear that unless the cause of illness in Americans was somehow determined and a concrete policy was drawn up to combat this trend, the situation could become financially unsustainable. From that sense of impending crisis, a special committee in the Senate was established, chaired by Senator George S. McGovern.

With top medical and nutritional specialists of the time, members of the committee collected food and health data from all over the world and studied the causes of increase in illnesses. The results and data were compiled in the 5,000-page McGovern Report.

Because the report concluded that many diseases were caused by wrong dietary habits, publication of this report forced Americans to make a big decision. There would be no way for Americans to become healthy unless their current dietary habits changed.

At that time in the U.S., a high-protein, high-fat diet, such as thick cuts of steak or high-fat hamburger meat for dinner, was fairly common. Proteins are indeed valuable because they are the basic element for building the body. For that reason, eating food rich in animal protein was thought to be good, not only for athletes and growing children, but also for the physically weak and elderly. Even in Japan, the deep-rooted idea that "meat is the source of stamina" was influenced by American dietary habits.

The McGovern Report not only refuted that common belief, but it also described the ideal diet as none other than the Japanese diet during Japan's "Genroku Period" (1688-1703), which consisted of grains as the staple food with side dishes such as seasonal vegetables, sea vegetables, and small amounts of small fish for protein. Because of this, the health benefits of Japanese food began to attract attention worldwide.

The common belief that if you do not eat meat, your muscles will not develop is demonstrably untrue. As proof of this, just take a look at nature. One would think that lions, being carnivores, would have extraordinary muscles. However, in reality, herbivores, like horses and deer, have much better developed muscles than lions. As proof of this, lions and tigers lack the stamina to pursue their prey for an extended period of time. They instead leap into action in an instant and use their speed to catch and kill their prey as quickly as possible. They do this because they themselves know that when it comes to endurance, they are no match for the better developed muscles of herbivores.

It is also untrue when we are told that we will not grow taller if we do not eat meat. Elephants and giraffes are several times taller than lions and tigers, but they are herbivores.

Eating meat does accelerate growth, and the rapid growth and maturation of children in the past few decades may be attributable to an increased intake of animal protein. Nevertheless, there is also a dangerous trap in eating meat. Once you reach a certain age, your body's growth changes into a phenomenon called aging. Eating meat may accelerate growth, but it will also speed up the aging process.

Perhaps you are not willing to cut back on eating meat. That does not change the fact that meat has a harmful effect on your health and speeds up the aging process. Before you close your mind (and this book), read the material that follows.

6 Reasons Why High Protein Diets Will Harm Your Health:

1. Toxins from meat breed cancer cells.

Each cell contains DNA (deoxyribonucleic acid), a chemical that contains the map for the body and its functions. The toxic byproducts of excessive animal fat and protein digestion can damage the DNA, turning the cells cancerous. The cancerous cells start multiplying on their own. Our blood contains red blood cells, white blood cells and lymphocytes. White cells and lymphocytes attack enemies such as bacteria and viruses, destroying them or rendering them harmless. When these cells are damaged this front line defense mechanism of the body malfunctions, and this can result in infection and the appearance of abnormal, cancerous cells.

2. Proteins Cause Allergic Reactions.

Proteins that have not been broken down into nutrients enter the blood stream as a foreign substance through the wall of the intestines. This often happens with small children. The body reacts to it as a foreign substance, creating an allergic reaction. This kind of protein allergy is most commonly caused by milk and eggs. Excessive intake of animal proteins and resultant allergic reactions are the cause of increasing incidences of atropic dermatitis, hives, collagen diseases, ulcerative colitis and Crohn's disease.

3. Excess Protein Stresses Liver and Kidneys.

Excess protein in the body must be broken down and eliminated through urine and causes a great burden on the liver and kidneys.

4. **Excessive Intake of Protein Causes Calcium Deficiency and Osteoporosis.**

When large amounts of amino acids are created, the blood becomes acidic, requiring calcium to neutralize it. Thus, excess protein consumption results in the loss of calcium. In addition, the phosphorus level in meat is very high and the blood must maintain a calcium to phosphorus ratio of between 1:1 and 1:2. A diet that increases the level of phosphorus will cause the body to draw calcium from teeth and bones to maintain the balance. Also, when one has lots of phosphorus and calcium in the body, phosphorus and calcium bind, producing calcium phosphate. The body cannot absorb this compound so it is excreted, adding to further loss of calcium, making the body susceptible to osteoporosis. This is why many people in countries with diets rich in animal proteins suffer from osteoporosis: porous bones result from a depletion of calcium.

5. **Excess Protein Can Result in a Lack of Energy.**

A great amount of energy is required to digest food. Excess protein is not completely metabolized and therefore not absorbed, leading to putrefaction in the intestines and the creation of toxic byproducts. A great amount of energy is demanded to detoxify these substances. When a large amount of energy is used a large number of free radicals are created. Free radicals are responsible for the aging process, cancer, heart disease and atherosclerosis.

6. **Excess Protein May Contribute to ADHD in Children.**

Studies in recent years show an increase in children with short attention spans who are prone to angry outbursts. Food and nutrition can have a significant impact on a child's behavior and social adaptability. There is a growing tendency for children at home and at school to consume large amounts of processed foods. Not only do these foods contain several additives, but processed foods tend to make the body acidic. Animal protein and refined sugar are also consumed in increased amounts while vegetables are often avoided. Animal protein and sugar demand increased calcium and magnesium leading to calcium deficiency. Calcium deficiency irritates the nervous system contributing to nervousness and irritability.

What Your Stomach and Intestines Can Tell You

In Japan, there is a concept that you can literally read in a person's facial features the quality of that person's life. In the United States, the saying goes, "It's written all over his face." Just as someone's facial features can be good or bad depending on the person's experiences and state of mind, the stomach and intestine also have good and bad characteristics that depict a person's health condition.

A healthy person's gastrointestinal characteristics are very clean. A healthy stomach is one in which the mucous membrane is uniformly pink without any bumps or irregularities on the surface, and blood vessels under the mucous are not visible. Furthermore, since a healthy person's mucous is transparent, it appears shiny when reflecting light from the endoscope. A healthy person's intestine is pink, extremely soft and has big, uniform folds.

Everybody has clean gastrointestinal characteristics as a child, but those features change depending on the person's daily diet and lifestyle.

An unhealthy person's stomach is spotty and, in certain areas, red and swollen. Moreover, when the stomach develops chronic or acute inflammation of the mucous membrane, which is prevalent among Americans and Japanese people alike, the stomach lining becomes thin and blood vessels are visible underneath the mucous membrane.

Furthermore, when the gastric mucosa begin to atrophy or shrivel up, the surface cells try to compensate by multiplying in certain areas, causing the gastric wall to become bumpy. At that point, it is just one step short to becoming cancerous. In an unhealthy intestine, because the muscles of the intestinal walls become thick and firm, unequal folds develop, causing constrictions in certain areas, as if rubber bands were squeezing it.

People with "dormant illnesses" who have not yet developed pain or physical ailments, might have little motivation to cut down on eating meat. Perhaps very few red-blooded Americans will heed my advice. Why? Perhaps because they cannot give up meat. Social pressures are too great. Maybe they've been relying on meat to make a meal for their entire lives and do not know what else to eat. However, the reason may also be that they cannot see what things look like inside their own gut.

When the exterior of our bodies start showing physical change, we tend to take the changes more seriously. Balding, wrinkles, fat, or sagging skin upset people and motivate them to spend time and money trying to treat these conditions. When it comes to changes within the digestive tract, out of sight is out of mind. People tend to think that unless they have a severe pain in the belly, everything must be fine in there. Nothing is done to take care of the inside of the stomach and intestines, and they continue to deteriorate. Later on, after people become sick, many regret not having made a lifestyle change to prevent the illness.

I myself am more concerned with the changes occurring inside the body than I am about those on the outside. In part, this is because I can *see* the interior characteristics through my colonoscope. Mainly, however, it is because I know that these internal changes are directly related to the person's overall health.

My patients who seriously follow the Enzyme Factor Diet and Lifestyle do so because they know their lives depend on it. For those who have previously had cancer, however, a healthy lifestyle that has a track record of producing a 0% recurrence rate usually takes precedence over everything else. But I would like to change this from 0% cancer recurrence rate to a 0% illness rate by having people with dormant illnesses follow this healthy lifestyle.

In order for that to happen, everyone must clearly understand what changes are occurring inside their intestines when they continue eating meat.

The biggest reason eating meat damages our intestines is because meat contains no dietary fiber but does contain a large amount of fat and cholesterol. In addition, meat causes the walls of the colon to gradually become thicker and firmer. This happens because the lack of dietary fiber in meat results in a significant decrease of stool in the colon, making the colon work harder than usual to excrete the small amount of stool through peristalsis. In other words, excessive peristaltic motion causes intestinal wall muscles to become thicker and bigger, making the colon firmer and shorter.

As the colonic walls become thicker, the lumen, or colonic cavity narrows. Although the internal pressure in the firm and narrow colon rises, when large amounts of fat are absorbed in addition to the animal protein, the layer of fat around the colon thickens, putting more pressure on the intestinal wall. And as this internal pressure in the colon rises, the mucous membrane gets pushed out from the inside, forming pocket-like cavities called "diverticuli" in a condition called "diverticulosis."

Now, the normally small amount of stool becomes even more difficult to push through the colon. As a result, the colon accumulates stagnant stool (impacted feces), which remain stagnant inside the colon for a long time. The stagnant stool accumulates as if clinging to the colon walls and, combined with diverticulosis, the stagnant stool goes into the pocket-like cavities, making excretion even more difficult.

Stagnant stool that accumulates in the diverticuli, or in between the folds, produces toxins, causing genetic mutations of cells in those sections and resulting in polyps. The polyps grow and can eventually become cancerous.

THE DIFFERENCE BETWEEN AMERICAN INTESTINES
AND JAPANESE INTESTINES

I first came to New York as a surgical resident in 1963. At that time, the typical method of examining colons was by barium enema, a procedure in which the colon was injected with barium, then examined by x-ray. Although this method could reveal whether or not there was a large polyp, it could not tell the minute details or internal condition of the colon. Moreover, a laparotomy—a large incision into the abdomen—was necessary in order to remove the polyp that was detected. Having a laparotomy meant placing a big burden on the patient, mentally and physically. Furthermore, with this method of examination, you could not tell whether the polyp was benign or cancerous until the surgeon actually looked inside the colon during surgery.

There existed an endoscope called a proctoscope at the time, but it was a straight metallic pipe-like tube, and no matter how hard they tried, examining doctors could only see about 20 cm from the anus.

Therefore, in 1967, I purchased an esophagoscope (used for examining the esophagus) that was made in Japan and discovered a way to use that fiberglass scope to examine the colon. That was my first colonoscope.

Afterwards, when a long scope (185cm) specifically for colon examination was developed, I purchased it and used it to examine my patients. When I looked at an American person's colon for the first time, I was surprised at how bad its condition was.

With a diet of meat, American colons were clearly firmer and shorter than Japanese colons. In addition to the lumen being narrower, ring-like bumps had formed in certain areas as though they were tied off with rubber bands. There were also many diverticuli and frequent accumulations of stagnant stool.

Such deterioration of intestinal conditions results not only in diseases like colon cancer, colonic polyps, and diverticulosis. Many people with unhealthy intestines in fact become ill with lifestyle-related diseases, such as fibroids, hypertension (high blood pressure), arteriosclerosis (hardening of the arteries), heart disease, obesity, breast cancer, prostate cancer and diabetes. When your intestines are unhealthy, your body is gradually weakened from the inside.

Many Americans had problems with their colons and, back then, it was said that one out of ten people had polyps. In fact, in the surgical department where I was a resident, surgeries for colonic polyp excisions constituted about one-third of all surgeries. The situation was such that laparotomies were being performed every day just to remove tiny polyps measuring 1-2 cm. This led me to wonder whether there was a way to remove polyps without placing such a heavy burden on patients.

Meanwhile, at that time in Japan, a "gastrocamera fiberscope" made of fiberglass with a camera lens attached to its tip was being put into practical use. So, in June of 1968, I made a momentous request to a Japanese manufacturer. I asked them to devise a wire that could be inserted into a colonoscope and used to burn off polyps without cutting open the abdomen. In 1969, after consulting many times with that company's office in New York and much testing, I became the first person in the world to succeed in performing a polypectomy — i.e., removing a polyp using a snare wire via a colonoscope without cutting open the abdomen.

This technological innovation was then applied to polyp excisions for the stomach, esophagus, and small intestine. After my cases of colonoscopic polypectomies were reported at the New York Surgical Society Conference in 1970 and the American Gastrointestinal Endoscopy Conference in 1971, a new surgical field called "surgical endoscopy" was established.

More than 30 years have passed since then. During this time, as I have continued to work in both the U.S. and Japan, I have observed changes in the gastrointestinal characteristics of people in both countries.

As Japan entered the 1960s and approached the period of rapid growth, that country learned to catch up and surpass America in many things.

Beginning about 1961 when milk was introduced in school lunches in Japan, people began eating dairy products such as cheese and yogurt on a daily basis. At the same time, vegetables and fish, which used to be the center of Japanese meals, began to be replaced by animal proteins, gradually transforming the Japanese diet into a high protein, high fat diet centered on hamburgers, steaks, and fried chicken. This trend has continued to this day.

In contrast, after publication of the 1977 McGovern Report, many Americans began focusing on improving their diet. These differences are evident in the intestinal characteristics of people in both the U.S. and Japan.

Steadily declining now because of changes in dietary habits, the once clean, healthy intestines of Japanese people now closely resemble the intestines of Americans who eat a diet centered on meat. On the other hand, many Americans who seriously thought about their health and reformed their high protein-high fat diet markedly improved their intestinal characteristics. As a result, since 1990, the rate of colonic polyps and cancers in America has been declining—clear evidence that you can promote intestinal health by improving your dietary habits.

THE STOMACH CANCER RATE IN JAPAN IS TENFOLD THAT OF AMERICA

Because of America's historical and cultural emphasis on eating meat, the intestinal characteristics of Americans remain generally worse than those in Japan. However, the stomachs of many Japanese are in fact much worse than those of Americans. Having examined the stomachs of both Americans and Japanese, I have found that Japanese people are twenty times more likely to have atrophic gastritis, a condition in which the stomach mucosa becomes thin. Moreover, because atrophic gastritis increases the chances of stomach cancer, the rate of stomach cancer is ten times higher in Japan than in America.

In both America and Japan, obesity is currently a big problem. However, there are not many Japanese who are as obese as their American counterparts. The fact is, Japanese people are incapable of becoming that obese. You can even see this in sumo wrestling, where it is the sumo wrestler's duty to gain weight. There are no Japanese sumo wrestlers with a body like that of Konishiki (a Hawaiian-born American sumo wrestler who weighed over 600 pounds and rose to the second highest rank of ozeki in Japanese sumo).

The Japanese cannot become as obese as Americans because before they reach that point, the Japanese develop stomach problems, preventing them from eating more. In other words, the reason Americans are able to become much bigger than the Japanese is that their digestive systems are stronger.

While examining stomachs using the endoscope, I found considerable differences between Japanese and Americans when it comes to the way they experience their symptoms. When I examine Japanese people, even though their condition may not be too serious, they complain about having stomach pains, feeling a great deal of discomfort, and heartburn. Interestingly, I discovered that Americans, even if their stomach or esophageal mucosa is considerably inflamed, will rarely complain as much as the Japanese about heartburn or other problems.

One reason such differences occur is the amount of vitamin A found in American food. Vitamin A protects not only the stomach mucosa, but all mucous membranes, such as those of the eye and trachea. Oil contains a lot of vitamin A. One could say that Japan's diet has become more westernized, but the volume of foods such as oil, butter and eggs that Japanese consume is much lower than the volume that Americans consume. If you think about the health of your entire body, these types of food are not good for you. But if you think only in terms of protecting mucous membranes throughout your body, they have some positive effects.

One other possibility regarding why Americans have stronger

gastrointestinal systems is the number of digestive enzymes their bodies contain. Digestive enzymes break down food and help the body absorb nutrients. The number of digestive enzymes determines the digestion and absorption of food. Digestion and absorption advance step-by-step as various digestive enzymes are released at each level of digestion. These levels start with saliva and move on to the stomach, duodenum, pancreas and small intestine. Under these circumstances, if each organ secretes enough digestive enzymes, then digestion and absorption will progress smoothly. However if an insufficient amount of digestive enzymes is secreted, then it will cause indigestion and put greater burden on the rest of the organs.

The reason many Japanese people easily feel symptoms like stomach pain or discomfort, even though their stomach condition may not be bad, is that they originally have a lower number of digestive enzymes than Americans.

Furthermore, Japanese people tend to immediately take stomach medication when their stomach conditions worsen, whereas many Americans do not. What Americans do take, however, are digestive enzyme supplements. But these supplements are not sold on the market in Japan, being available only by prescription when the doctor deems it necessary. In America, digestive enzymes are extremely popular supplements. They can easily be purchased in health food stores and supermarkets.

The fact is, taking medication to suppress the secretion of stomach acid further accelerates the deterioration of the stomach lining. Highly popular antacids and stomach medications like the combination of H2 blockers and proton-pump inhibitors are advertised as being highly effective in suppressing the secretion of stomach acid. However, if stomach acid is suppressed with medication, the gastric mucosa atrophies, and the result is what I have already discussed earlier; namely, gastric mucosal atrophy progresses, and this condition may lead to the development of stomach cancer.

If you have stomach pain or discomfort, please tell your doctor exactly what your physical conditions are and then have him or her prescribe the appropriate enzyme supplements according to your symptoms. Or, shop for them in a health foods store, reading labels carefully. By taking digestive enzyme supplements, your stomach conditions will markedly improve.

THE MORE ANTACIDS YOU TAKE, THE WORSE YOUR STOMACH WILL BE

There are two places in the human body where an extremely strong acidic environment serves as a protective measure. One is the stomach, and the other is the female vagina. These two places both have strong acid levels of pH 1.5 to 3.0, the main function being to kill bacteria.

Whether you are taking a bath or having sex, bacteria enters the vagina, and strong acids are produced by the lactobacilli in the vagina that kill invading bacteria.

Bacteria enter the stomach when you consume food. It is estimated that as many as 300 billion to 400 billion bacteria enter the stomach with each meal. The strong acid found in gastric juices kills most of these bacteria.

In other words, because bacteria invade both the stomach and the vagina, they must produce strong acid in order to kill the bacteria. Often when stomach acid, indispensable for protecting the body, is suppressed with medication bacteria with strong toxins pass through the stomach and into the intestines, where they can cause diarrhea and various illnesses.

If stomach acid secretion is suppressed, the secretion of pepsin and hydrochloric acid, which activate digestive enzymes, is also suppressed, resulting in indigestion. Moreover, insufficient stomach acid makes it more difficult to absorb iron and minerals such as calcium and magnesium. Thus, people who have had gastrectomies[1] for stomach ulcers or stomach

---

1   Removal of all or part of the stomach.

cancer are always anemic because, when their stomachs are surgically removed, they no longer secrete stomach acid and are unable to absorb iron.

Furthermore, suppressing stomach acid destroys the bacterial balance in the intestine, resulting in a weakening of the immune system. It is said that approximately 100 trillion bacteria of some 300 different varieties reside in the human intestine. Among them, there are so-called good bacteria like the lactobacillus bifidus (bifidobacterium) and bad bacteria such as the Welsh bacteria. The majority of bacteria in the intestine, however, are neither good nor bad, but intermediate bacteria. These intermediate bacteria have unique properties so that if the number of good bacteria in the intestine multiplies, these intermediate bacteria become good bacteria; whereas, if the number of bad bacteria multiplies, the intermediates then become bad bacteria. Thus, the intermediates tilt the balance between good and bad bacteria, and that balance determines the overall health of the intestinal environment.

If stomach acid secretion is insufficient, digestive enzymes cannot be activated, resulting in undigested food advancing straight into the intestines. Food that should have been primarily digested and absorbed in the intestine remains undigested in the colon. The temperature inside the human colon is 98.6°F, which is equivalent to midsummer heat. The undigested food decomposes and abnormal fermentation occurs. As a result, the number of bad bacteria multiplies abnormally in the colon, weakening the immune system.

In this way, the more antacids you take, the more damage your body suffers. To avoid this damage, you need to *prevent* heartburn or bloating sensations that make you want to take antacids. If you understand the cause of heartburn and bloating, you can prevent it with just a little precaution.

Heartburn occurs when stomach acids flow back into the esophagus. The esophagus is susceptible to acid because it is typically an alkaline environment. Thus, when stomach acid builds up in the esophagus, people unconsciously swallow their alkaline saliva, washing down stomach acid that had flowed up. However, when you overeat or experience indigestion, causing acid to build up and making it difficult for the acid to be washed down with saliva, it results in scratch-like sores called erosions in the esophagus. Under that situation, if stomach acid flows up to the esophagus, it is like rubbing alcohol on a wound, causing symptoms of pain or discomfort commonly known as heartburn. And the relief you feel after taking antacids comes from suppression of further stomach acid secretion.

In other words, in order to suppress heartburn, all you have to do is prevent things in the stomach from backing up into the esophagus. And in order to do that, you must first refrain from overeating and overdrinking and cut down on smoking, alcohol and coffee. Another important thing to remember is to finish eating dinner four or five hours before going to bed so that your stomach is empty when you go to sleep.

On the stomach mucosa, there are tiny projections called villi that secrete stomach acids. However, if one continues to take antacids in order to suppress the secretion of stomach acid, these villi become shorter and shorter, weakening their function. This is what is known as mucosal atrophy. As atrophy of the mucosa progresses, the gastric mucosa becomes thin, causing inflammation — atrophic gastritis. Stomachs with atrophic gastritis easily become a hotbed of Helicobacter pylon (H. pylon) and other types of bacteria, steadily worsening the inflammation of the stomach and, in the end, causing stomach cancer.

H. pylori infection is common in the United States and infected persons have a two- to six-fold increased risk of developing stomach cancer. H. Pylori can conceal themselves either inside mucosal cells or inside the mucus, which protects the gastric mucosa from stomach acids. Since H. pylon is contracted orally, the infection rate increases with age, and it is estimated that the H. pylori infection rate among people over the age of 50 is 50%.

Being infected with H. pylori does not always lead to stomach cancer, but in order to suppress the H. pylori from multiplying, it is better to avoid taking stomach medication including antacids as much as possible.

ALL DRUGS ARE ALIEN TO THE BODY

Americans take medicine too casually. Although it may be necessary to treat certain conditions, I believe that all drugs, prescription and non-prescription are basically harmful to the body over the long term. Some people believe that herbal medicines have no side effects and are only beneficial, but that is also a mistake. Whether chemical products or herbal medicine, it does not change the fact that medicine in general is alien to the body.

The last time I was sick was at age 19, when I came down with the flu, so I have hardly taken any medicine in my life. I am like the proverbial canary in the coal mine. Since I have not taken any medication for several decades, do not consume alcohol or tobacco, and eat only foods that do not contain agricultural chemicals or additives, I will have an extreme reaction to even a small amount of medicine whenever I take any. For example, if I drink miso soup containing chemical seasonings, my pulse rate increases by 20, and I can clearly feel my face becoming flushed. Even if I drink only one cup of coffee, my blood pressure increases by 10 to 20 points.

Nowadays, many people like myself who react to even small amounts of medicines are labeled "drug hypersensitive," but I consider this a complete misnomer. The human body is like this in its natural state. Since most people regularly consume alcohol, tobacco, caffeine and soft drinks, and eat meals that use food additives and chemical seasoning, their bodies build up a tolerance to chemical substances, thus becoming desensitized to stimulus.

However, since I am also a physician, I do on occasion prescribe medication to my patients when it seems necessary. As long as doctors continue to prescribe medication, they have the responsibility of at least choosing medicines that will put minimal burden on the body. For this reason, before I prescribed any new medication, I always used to test that medication on my own body, which reacts sensitively to drugs. This involved my taking 1/4 or 1/8 of the prescribed dosage and seeing my body's reaction. I verified the medicine's safety by experimenting with it on myself.

In America, of course, the widely known side effects of medicine are written in minute detail. Still, if I do not take it myself, I will never know the true effect of the drug. In fact, many types of medication produce reactions that are not detailed in their explanatory pamphlets. In this way, I could explain both my own experience and publicly known side effects to my patients, and only with their complete understanding do I prescribe the medicine to them.

In recent years, however, I have stopped using my own body to test the effects of medication, because a particular drug I tested on myself put me in a condition in which I thought I would die. That drug was a popular medication to treat erectile dysfunction in men.

At first, I tried to break the 50mg tablet, the smallest dosage available, down to 1/4 its size. However, the tablet is so hard that I could not break it, no matter how hard I tried. So then I shaved off a little bit of the drug, put the powder on my fingertip and licked it. Although the amount I took was probably not even 1/7 of the normal amount, the suffering I endured afterwards was excruciating. When I think about it now, I am really glad I did not take more.

The effects appeared in only about ten minutes. The first reaction I experienced was nasal congestion. Then, I began having difficulty breathing; my face started feeling as if it were swelling up. The breathing difficulty continued to worsen to the point that I thought I would just suffocate and die. To tell you the truth, getting an erection was the last thing on my mind. At that moment, experiencing such suffering and severe anxiety, I just prayed silently that I would not die on the spot.

What I learned from this was that the faster the effects of the drug appear, the stronger its toxicity. When choosing a medication, please do not forget that a highly effective drug which produces immediate relief will be that much more harmful to the body than many other medicines.

Even with gastrointestinal medication, there are quite a few unexpected side effects. For example, if a man regularly takes antacids like H2 blockers, there is a possibility that he may experience erectile dysfunction. There are also data showing a sharp decrease in sperm count. That is why it is not an exaggeration when I say the problems we have seen in recent years concerning male sterility can be attributed to the various strong antacids on the market.

Among people who are used to receiving prescription medication, there are some who probably do not know what medication they are taking or what the effects and side effects will be. But any kind of medicine will place some stress on the body, and thus, it is important to know exactly what the risks are.

HEARTBURN IS YOUR BODY'S WARNING; PAY ATTENTION

Over the years I have noticed that my breast cancer patients often have bad intestinal characteristics like diverticulosis and stagnant stool. It is believed that breast and colon cancer are generally unrelated. From what I've seen in my practice they are actually closely related.

Researchers are trying desperately to find the cause of cancer, but, in reality, it is not caused by just one factor. This is true for other illnesses as well, because various factors surrounding us – food, water, medicine, lack of exercise, stress, living environment – all intricately influence our bodies and lead to the development of illness.

Owing to the advancement of specialized fields of medical practice, there has been a tendency to look at only a particular area of the body where an illness develops. When patients complain of heartburn, many doctors tell them to take medicine to suppress the secretion of stomach acid because they believe the cause of heartburn is "gastric hyperacidity." In other words, they believe that too much stomach acid is being produced, and that this hypersecretion needs to be suppressed with medication.

It is true that if you suppress the secretion of stomach acid, the symptoms of heartburn disappear. But, as I have already discussed, this form of treatment will cause serious damage and put stress on all the other parts of the body. I think the idea that heartburn, acid reflux and acid indigestion are results of "gastric hyperacidity" is wrong. In fact, *there is no such thing as too much stomach acid*. Stomach acid is produced because it is necessary to maintain the balance and overall health of the body. By overriding such natural mechanisms of the body with medicine, I believe you only end up shortening your lifespan.

The human body consists of a very intricate system, delicately balanced. That system also functions inside each of the approximately 60 trillion cells that make up the human body. If you are serious about your health, think about your body starting at the cellular level.

Our cells are always being replaced by new cells. Cells in some areas of the body are completely replaced by new ones in several days, while in other areas the process can take as long as several years. Eventually, they all get replaced. These new cells are made from the water and food that we consume on a daily basis. Based on this, we can say that the quality of food and water we consume determines our health.

Our gastrointestinal system, which absorbs our food and water, is thus the foundation of our body. If the quality of food and water is bad, the gastrointestinal system is the first to suffer. Later, the bad elements that are absorbed get transported by blood vessels to all cells throughout the body. No matter how bad the ingredients, the cells can only use the transported material to make new cells. In this way, the quality of food and water determines the health of the entire body.

After I discovered that gastrointestinal characteristics reflect the health condition of the entire body, I asked my patients to fill out questionnaires about their diet and lifestyle. This was so I could learn what is good and bad for the body without influence from any "common knowledge" I had until then. I could reach my own conclusions by observing my clinical results. What happens inside the human body is different from what happens in a laboratory experiment. The only way to discover the truth is by asking your body directly.

THE NUMBER OF ENZYMES IS THE KEY TO YOUR HEALTH

As I collated the results from my questionnaire and various clinical data, I found there is one factor playing a central role in maintaining a person's health. That factor is the enzyme factor.

As mentioned earlier, "enzyme" is a general term for "a protein catalyst made within the cells of a living thing." Simply put, it is an element necessary for a living thing to live.

Whether animal or plant, wherever there is life, you will find enzymes. For example, a bud sprouts from a plant seed because enzymes are at work. Enzymes are also at work when a bud grows into a leaf. Our body's activities are also supported by many enzymes. Digestion and absorption, the metabolism of old cells being replaced by new cells, the breakdown of toxins and detoxification are all a result of enzyme functions.

Of the more than 5,000 types of enzymes working in the human body there are two broad categories: those made inside the body and those coming from outside in the form of food. Among enzymes made in the body, about 3,000 kinds are made by intestinal bacteria.

One commonality among people with good gastrointestinal characteristics is that they eat a lot of fresh foods containing many enzymes. This not only means consuming enzymes from the outside, but also creating an intestinal environment conducive to intestinal bacteria's actively producing enzymes.

On the other hand, the things people with bad gastrointestinal characteristics and features have in common are lifestyle habits that accelerate the exhaustion of enzymes. Habitual use of alcohol and tobacco, overeating, eating food containing food additives, stressful environments, and use of medicine all exhaust large numbers of enzymes. Other things that consume large quantities of enzymes include eating bad food that produces toxins inside the colon, being exposed to ultraviolet rays and electromagnetic waves that produce free radicals, requiring detoxification by enzymes, and emotional stress.

What we learn from this is that it is necessary to develop a lifestyle that increases rather than uses up your body's enzymes. This has become the basis for the Enzyme Factor Diet and Lifestyle.

If a body possesses abundant enzymes, its life energy and immune system are heightened. Avoid exhaustion of your body's enzymes—maintain a sufficient level of enzymes—and your body will be healthy.

At present, a living body is the only thing that can make enzymes. Although we can artificially make foods containing enzymes, like fermented foods, microorganisms such as bacteria are the ones actually making those enzymes. Thus, even if we can create an environment where microorganisms make enzymes, we cannot artificially synthesize and make enzymes ourselves.

This is why The Enzyme Factor Diet and Lifestyle emphasizes the importance of food. As I have stated before, eating foods containing enzymes creates an intestinal environment that allows intestinal bacteria to produce enzymes. If every living thing has a predetermined enzyme potential, it becomes even more vital for us, living in today's stressful and polluted environments, to consume and efficiently use enzymes made by other living things.

It All Comes Down to Source Enzymes

Although I have talked about "enzymes" as a single word, more than 5,000 types of enzymes are needed in order for people to conduct their life activities. Many types exist because each enzyme has only one function.

For example, the digestive enzyme amylase, which is found in saliva, will react only to starch, while pepsin, found in gastric juice, reacts only to protein.

If you think about it in this way, one question presents itself. That is, no matter how much we supplement our body's enzymes with food and intestinal bacteria, how can we be sure we are consuming the "right kind" of enzyme, the type that is needed by our body at a given time?

The fact is, even if you eat foods abundant in enzymes, those enzymes are not usually absorbed and used by the human body directly. Some enzymes, like the ones in daikon radish and yams, work directly in digestive organs such as the mouth and stomach. But those are exceptions. Most food enzymes are broken down by the process of digestion and absorbed through the intestine as peptides or amino acids.

You may wonder why these enzymes are important if you cannot absorb and utilize them directly. But that is not the point. The clinical data I have collected clearly show that people whose diets are abundant in enzymes also have a high level of body enzymes.

So what is happening in the body to produce these enzymes? From this point I will explain my theory, based on over forty years in daily medical practice, examining hundreds of thousands of digestive tracts. Observing my clinical data, I developed a theory that there must be an enzyme prototype — a source enzyme — what I like to call the "miracle" enzyme.

I began thinking there might be an enzyme prototype because I noticed that when a large amount of a specific enzyme is used in a particular area of the body, there appeared a shortage of necessary enzymes in other parts of the body. One example of this, which I earlier stated, is when a large quantity of alcohol is consumed, a large number of enzymes are used to break down the alcohol, resulting in a shortage of enzymes necessary for digestion and absorption in other areas.

From this observation, I reached the conclusion that the several thousand kinds of enzymes must all originate from a prototype, which is made first and, in response to a specific need, gets converted to a specific enzyme and used where it is needed.

Enzymes are responsible for all functions of a living body. The movement of your fingers, your breathing and your heart beating are all activities made possible by the work of enzymes. But the system would be inefficient if each enzyme used for a particular activity is produced from the start in its final form, without respect to the body's changing needs.

If my theory is correct, when one organ or part of the body uses an excessive amount of its enzyme supply, the body will have a difficult time maintaining homeostasis, repairing cells, and supporting the nervous, endocrine, and immune systems, because it will deplete the source enzymes and thus create a shortage of enzymes in those other areas.

The other reason I believe in the existence of source enzymes is that habitual use of alcohol, tobacco, or drugs, will cause your body to develop a tolerance for these substances.

For example, if you drink alcohol, it is absorbed in the stomach and intestine, accumulates in the liver, and gets broken down by enzymes specifically for alcohol. There are several kinds of enzymes working in the liver for this purpose. However, the rate of breaking down alcohol differs considerably from person to person. People with fast alcohol metabolism possess many enzymes that are available to break down the alcohol in the liver. Such people have a high alcohol tolerance level. On the other hand, people with low tolerance for alcohol have too few enzymes available to break the alcohol down.

However, even people who initially had low tolerance to alcohol can raise the tolerance and eventually be able to drink a lot. When the liver recognizes that a large number of enzymes are needed, the body adjusts itself to concentrate its enzymes on alcohol metabolism.

In this way, the number of enzymes in a particular area of the body changes when necessary. And what makes this possible? It is the existence of the source enzyme, which can become any type of enzyme. When foods containing enzymes are consumed, source enzymes get stored in the body, ready for use when the need arises.

At present, the existence of a source enzyme is still a theory, but I have supporting evidence from the clinical data I have collected.

Why Anti-Cancer Drugs Do Not Cure Cancer

I have already talked about the harm drugs tend to exert on the body. The biggest problem is that drugs exhaust large numbers of source enzymes. Of all drugs, the most challenging ones for source enzymes are anticancer drugs.

Under current medical practice, chemotherapy drugs are used for a short period of time following cancer surgery to prevent the cancer's spread, even if there is no evidence of the cancer's having metastasized. They work by poisoning many cells of the body, normal as well as malignant, in the hopes that the body will regenerate the normal cells while all abnormal ones, the malignant ones, will die off completely.

Since chemotherapy drugs are deadly poisons, I will not use them in any but the most extraordinary situations. For example, even if cancer is found outside the colon in the lymph nodes, I will not use chemotherapy. My treatment plan consists of first surgically removing the part invaded by cancer, and, once that visible cancer is removed, I then begin to eliminate what I believe may be the *cause* of cancer in that patient. Needless to say, I first have them abstain from tobacco and alcohol and completely stop consuming meat, milk and dairy products. Along with following the Enzyme Factor Diet and Lifestyle, I also have them adjust their mental perspective, training their minds to conjure as many happy thoughts and feelings as possible. In this way, my treatment plan aims to prevent the recurrence of cancer by heightening the body's immunity through better physical and mental health.

Enzymes are responsible for cell repair and regeneration, maintaining the immune system and other life activities. The number of source enzymes in the body determines whether or not the immune system functions properly.

I consider anticancer drugs such as chemotherapy poisonous because when they enter the body, they release large amounts of highly toxic free radicals. By doing this, the drugs kill cancer cells in the entire body.

However, cancer cells are not the only thing they kill. Many normal cells also die in the process. The old saying "fight fire with fire" probably shapes the way doctors who use anticancer drugs pursue their work. At the same time, chemotherapy drugs can also be considered carcinogenic.

At all times, the human body is working to maintain homeostasis. That is why when large amounts of highly toxic free radicals accumulate in the body, source enzymes throughout the body transform into enzymes that detoxify those free radicals. The body tries its best to neutralize the biggest damage caused by free radicals.

To be sure, there have been many people who have overcome cancer with chemotherapy, but many of these people are young and have most likely retained most of their source enzymes. The levels of source enzymes decrease with age. Of course, there are individual differences, but chemo is more likely to work in young people because there are still enough source enzymes left to help the body recover from the stress of the treatment.

The well-known side effects of chemotherapy are appetite loss, nausea, and loss of hair, but I believe all those symptoms occur because large amounts of source enzymes are being used for detoxification. The number of source enzymes consumed in the detoxification process after chemo would have to be enormous.

When there are not enough digestive enzymes, a person experiences appetite loss. At the same time, cell metabolism slows down because of insufficient metabolic enzymes and the mucous membrane of the stomach and intestine becomes irregular, causing nausea. Metabolic enzyme deficiency leads to flaky skin, nail breaks and loss of hair. (Although there is a difference in the level of severity, the same thing happens when other kinds of medicine enter the body.)

Drugs cannot fundamentally cure diseases. The only fundamental path to a cure for any illness lies in our daily lifestyle.

WHY THERE IS NO RELAPSE OF CANCER FOR PEOPLE FOLLOWING THE ENZYME FACTOR DIET AND LIFESTYLE

Tumors form when abnormal cells multiply and become tissue masses. They can be benign tumors, not metastasizing or infiltrating other parts of the body, with limited growth. Or, they can be invasive, malignant tumors — cancer.

When diagnosed with cancer, the first thing you worry about is whether or not the cancer has metastasized. If it has, it becomes difficult to surgically remove all of the affected areas and still have a complete recovery.

Metastasis means the appearance of cancer in a region other than where the cancer first developed. In general, cancer is said to metastasize when the cancerous cells travel through lymph nodes and blood vessels to other organs, where they then multiply. But my thinking on this is slightly different. I believe that just the process of cancer cells multiplying in one place has repercussions in other organs, making the entire body more cancer-prone.

Usually, cancer is first discovered when the tumor has grown to a diameter of at least one centimeter. A tumor develops from one cancerous cell that multiplies. It requires several hundred million cells to form a tumor.

Therefore, it takes more than a short time to form a tumor. Cancer is a lifestyle-related disease. Thus, the appearance of cancer somewhere means that most likely there are cancerous cells that have not yet grown into a tumor in other parts of the body. These cells are like a series of time bombs planted throughout your body. What determines which of those bombs will explode first are such factors as the person's hereditary characteristics and living environment. For someone who eats a lot of food containing agricultural chemicals and food additives, the liver, which controls the detoxification process, might be the site where a bomb explodes first. For people who have irregular meal times and drink tea or take antacids on a regular basis, the bombs in their stomachs may explode first. Even if the lifestyle is the same, the location where the first bomb explodes may differ depending on hereditary factors. In other words, cancer is not a localized disease that invades only one area of the body. It is a full body disease that affects the body as a whole.

The reason cancer appears to spread or metastasize everywhere is because the bombs planted throughout the body explode one after another with a time lag. Considering this, it becomes questionable whether surgically removing the primary diseased area, including the lymph nodes and blood vessels, is truly the correct approach.

It is considered dangerous to surgically remove cancer from its primary site if you overlook the metastasis, since the removal will accelerate growth of the metastasized cancer in other parts of the body. However, that is only natural if you think of cancer as a full body disease. If you remove organs, lymph nodes and blood vessels from a body already low on energy, it is only natural that the body's immune functions will deteriorate even more rapidly.

In cases of colon cancer, I do not remove the messentary[2] to prevent the spread of cancer to the lymph nodes or other areas. I believe more damage is done by losing the lymph nodes than by leaving a little cancer intact.

In modern medicine, it is thought that unless cancer is surgically removed, the diseased organ will not heal on its own. But that has not been my experience. The immune system and natural healing strength of humans seem to be more powerful than commonly believed. As proof of this, my patients who still have a little cancer left in their lymph nodes but follow my dietary therapy experience no recurrence of cancer.

If you improve your diet by following the Enzyme Factor Diet and Lifestyle, source enzymes, which are life's energy, will be supplemented in large quantities. At the same time, lifestyle habits that exhaust source

---

2   Any of several folds of the peritoneum that connect the intestines to the dorsal abdominal wall.

enzymes are corrected, so there are twin benefits. The number of source enzymes is sufficiently restored, strengthening the body's potential immune power and activating immune cells to suppress the recurrence of cancer.

There is a limit to this therapy. If the cancer has already progressed to the last stage, no matter how much you improve your diet or lifestyle or are given supplements to boost your immune system, it would be difficult to completely restore your body's normal functions. That is because the source enzymes have already been exhausted.

However, in my clinical experience, even people who have one-third to one-half of the inner circumference of their colon invaded by cancer would have no recurrence of cancer and could restore their health *if*, after the original cancer has been removed, they followed the proper diet and eating habits and took supplements instead of chemotherapy, to enable their source enzymes to work more efficiently.

Most of my patients primarily come for routine examinations, so I do not examine many patients with advanced cancer. However, of those cancer patients who practice the Enzyme Factor Diet and Lifestyle following surgery, not one of them has had any recurrence or metastasis. This fact deserves close attention.

THE LIMITED VALUE OF DRUGS

Again, on the most fundamental level, most drugs do not cure diseases. Drugs can be useful when there is severe pain or bleeding or in emergencies to suppress symptoms that must be alleviated. Even I sometimes prescribe H2 blockers like antacids to patients who complain of bleeding or pain from stomach ulcers. But I advise my patients to refrain from taking such medication longer than 2-3 weeks. While the pain is being alleviated by the medication, the cause of the ulcer is removed. There are various causes of ulcers, such as stress and the amount, quality, or time of meals, and unless those root causes are dealt with, no amount of medicine will be effective in curing the condition. Even though it may appear as if the ulcer has been temporarily cured with medication, it will certainly flare up again.

The only fundamental path to a cure for any illness lies in our daily lifestyle. Therefore, once the cause is removed and the stomach ulcer is healed, in order to prevent the ulcer from ever occurring again, it is important to follow the proper dietary habits regularly.

Source enzymes are not produced automatically. When you are careful about eating properly and living a healthy lifestyle that does not waste enzymes, that is when life itself produces the energy your body needs. Knowing how to limit the unnecessary depletion of your precious source enzymes is the secret to curing illnesses and living a long and healthy life.

DIETARY COMMON SENSE CAN BE
HAZARDOUS TO YOUR BODY

If we reexamine what we thought was common sense regarding food and digestion, we see that many things that we commonly consider good for the body actually work against the body's natural mechanisms.

Take, for example, meals thought to be good for sick people. Chicken soup is a favorite sick-person food in the United States. Bland foods, like white bread and pudding, are considered good for ulcer patients. If you are hospitalized in Japan, no matter what your condition, the hospital will immediately feed you rice porridge. Hospitals believe they are being considerate to their patients, especially those who have had internal surgery, by telling them, "Let's start you off with some rice porridge so we don't put too much stress on your stomach and intestines." But this is a big mistake.

I give my patients regular meals from the start, even if they have had stomach surgery. If you know how enzymes work, then you will understand immediately why unprocessed food is better than porridge.

It is better because it requires you to chew well. Chewing stimulates the secretion of saliva. Digestive enzymes found in saliva, when mixed with food while chewing, improve digestion and absorption because the breakdown of food progresses smoothly. However, porridge is soft to begin with, so it gets swallowed without being chewed well. Porridge does not digest well because not enough enzymes have been mixed in, whereas normal food that is chewed well also digests well.

I have even served regular sushi for lunch to patients three days after they have had stomach surgery. But then, I instruct them to properly "chew each mouthful 70 times." Chewing well is very important, and not just for sick people. In order to carry out the digestion and absorption process smoothly, I advise people, even those without any gastrointestinal problems, to consciously chew 30–50 times per mouthful at every meal.

The other mistake often seen with hospital food is milk. The main nutrients found in milk are protein, fat, glucose, calcium and vitamins. Milk is very popular because it contains a lot of calcium and is supposed to prevent osteoporosis.

But the truth is, there is no other food that is as difficult to digest as milk. Since milk is a smooth liquid substance, there are some people who drink it like water when they are thirsty, but that is a big mistake. Casein, which accounts for approximately 80% of the protein found in milk, immediately clumps together once it enters the stomach, making digestion very difficult. Furthermore, that component is homogenized in the milk sold in stores. Homogenization means equalizing the fat content in milk by stirring it. The reason homogenization is bad is that when milk is stirred, air gets mixed in, turning the milk's fat component into an oxidized fatty substance — fat in an advanced state of oxidation. In other words, homogenized milk produces free radicals and exerts a very negative influence on the body.

The milk containing oxidized fat then gets pasteurized at high temperatures over 212°F. Enzymes are sensitive to heat, and begin to be destroyed at temperatures 200°F. In other words, milk sold in stores not only lacks precious enzymes, but the fat is oxidized and the quality of the proteins is changed due to the high temperature. In a sense, milk is the worst type of food.

In fact, I have heard that if you feed milk sold in stores to a calf instead of milk straight from the mother cow, the calf will die in four or five days. Life cannot be sustained with foods that do not have enzymes.

MILK CAUSES INFLAMMATION

The first time I learned how bad milk is for the body was more than 35 years ago, when my own children developed atopic dermatitis[3] at six or seven months of age.

The children's mother followed the pediatrician's instructions, but no matter how much treatment they received, the children's dermatitis did not improve at all. Then, at around age three or four, my son began having severe diarrhea. And finally, he even started getting blood in his stool. Upon examination with an endoscope, I discovered that the toddler manifested early stages of ulcerative colitis[4].

Knowing ulcerative colitis is closely linked to one's diet, I focused on what kind of food the children usually ate. As it turned out, just when the children began developing atopic dermatitis, my wife had stopped breastfeeding and had started giving them milk under the pediatrician's advice. We eliminated all milk and milk products from the children's diet from that point on. Sure enough, the bloody stool and diarrhea, even the atopic dermatitis, completely subsided.

Following that experience, I began obtaining an itemized list of how much milk and milk products were consumed when I asked my patients about their dietary history. According to my clinical data, there is a high likelihood of developing a predisposition to allergies by consuming milk and milk products. This correlates with recent allergy studies that report

---

3   A severe skin inflammation
4   Severe inflammation with ulcers on the inside of the colon

that when pregnant women drink milk, their children are more prone to develop atopic dermatitis.

During the past 30 years in Japan, the number of patients with atopic dermatitis and hay fever has increased at an astonishing rate. That number may currently be as much as one out of every five people. There are many theories as to why there has been such a rapid increase in the number of people with allergies, but I believe the number one cause is the introduction of milk in school lunches in the early 1960s.

Milk, which contains many oxidized fatty substances, damages the intestinal environment, increasing the amount of bad bacteria and destroying the balance of the intestinal bacterial flora. As a result, toxins such as free radicals, hydrogen sulfides, and ammonia are produced in the intestine. Research about what kind of process these toxins go through and what kinds of illnesses arise is still ongoing, but several research papers have reported that milk not only causes various allergies but is also linked with diabetes among children[5]. These research papers are available on the internet, so I encourage you to read them yourselves.

WHY DRINKING TOO MUCH MILK WILL CAUSE OSTEOPOROSIS

The biggest common misconception about milk is that it helps prevent osteoporosis. Since the calcium content in our bodies decreases with age, we are told to drink a lot of milk to prevent osteoporosis. But this is a big mistake. Drinking too much milk actually *causes* osteoporosis.

It is commonly believed that calcium in milk is better absorbed than the calcium in other foods such as small fish, but that is not entirely true.

The calcium concentration in human blood is normally fixed at 9-10 mg. However, when you drink milk, the calcium concentration in your blood suddenly rises. Although at first glance, it may seem as if a lot of calcium has been absorbed, this rise in blood calcium level has its

---

5   *See* www.sciencenews.org/pages/sn_arc99/6_26_99/fob2.htm

downside. When the calcium concentration in the blood suddenly rises, the body tries to return this abnormal level back to normal by excreting calcium from the kidneys through urine. In other words, if you try to drink milk in order to get calcium, this actually produces the ironic result of decreasing the overall level of calcium in your body. All of the four big dairy countries – America, Sweden, Denmark and Finland – where a lot of milk is consumed every day, see many cases of hip fractures and osteoporosis.

In contrast to this, small fish and seaweed, which Japanese people have been eating for ages and were originally thought to be low in calcium, contain calcium that is not quickly absorbed in a way that raises the blood calcium concentration level. Moreover, there were hardly any cases of osteoporosis in Japan during the time when people did not drink milk. Even now, you do not hear about many people having osteoporosis among those who do not drink milk on a regular basis. The body can absorb the necessary calcium and minerals through the digestion of small shrimp, fish, and seaweed.

Why I Question the "Myth" About Yogurt

Recently in Japan, various types of yogurt such as "Caspian Sea yogurt" and "aloe yogurt" have become very popular because of their widely advertised health benefits. But I believe these are all misrepresentations.

What I often hear from people who eat yogurt is that their gastrointestinal condition has improved, they are no longer constipated, or their waist has gotten smaller. And they believe these results are due to the lactobacilli found in all yogurts.

However, this belief in the benefits of lactobacilli is questionable from the start. Lactobacilli are originally found in the human intestine. These bacteria are called "intestinal resident bacteria." The human body has a defense system against bacteria and viruses coming from the outside, so even those bacteria that are normally good for your body, like lactobacilli, will be attacked and destroyed by the body's natural defenses if they are not intestinal resident bacteria.

The first line of defense is stomach acid. When lactobacilli from the yogurt enter the stomach, most are killed by stomach acid. For that reason, there have been recent improvements made and yogurts are being sold with the catchphrase, "lactobacilli that reach your intestine."

However, even if the bacteria do reach the intestine, is it really possible for them to work hand in hand with the intestinal resident bacteria?

The reason I question this claim about yogurt is because in the clinical setting, the intestinal characteristics of people who eat yogurt everyday are never good. I strongly suspect that, even if the lactobacilli in yogurt reach the intestine alive, they do not make the intestine work better but only disrupt the intestinal flora instead.

Then why do many people feel yogurt is effective in improving their health? For many, yogurt seems to "cure" constipation. This "cure," however, is actually a mild case of diarrhea. Here is the way this probably works: Adults lack enough of the enzyme that breaks down lactose. Lactose is the sugar found in milk products, but lactase, the enzyme that breaks down lactose, begins to decrease in our bodies as we grow older. This is natural in a sense, because milk is something infants drink, not adults. In other words, lactase is an enzyme that is not required by adults.

Yogurt contains a lot of lactose. Thus, when you eat yogurt, it cannot be properly digested owing to the lack of lactase enzymes, which in turn results in indigestion. In short, many people develop mild diarrhea when they eat yogurt. Consequently, this mild diarrhea, which is really the excretion of stagnant stool that has been accumulating in the colon until then, gets mistakenly characterized as a cure for constipation.

Your intestine's condition will worsen if you eat yogurt everyday. I can say this with confidence based on my clinical observations. If you eat yogurt everyday, the smell of your stool and gas should be increasingly pungent. This is an indication that your intestinal environment is getting worse. The reason for the smell is that toxins are being produced inside the colon. Thus, even though people talk about the health effects of yogurt in general (and yogurt companies are more than pleased to tout their own products), in reality, there are many things about yogurt that are not good for your body.

As I stated in the beginning, we have now entered an age where we need to look out for our own health. Instead of just accepting information someone gives you, it is necessary to ascertain the truth by testing the information with your own body.

When I say you must test with your own body, I do not mean just by eating or trying something else. The person who believed yogurt cleared up constipation because it gave her diarrhea was not looking at the whole picture. Testing with your own body means first getting the best advice you can, then practicing it, and finally having your gastrointestinal tract examined periodically by a trusted doctor. This will allow you to confirm or reject the results of other people's advice. If you plan to practice the Enzyme Factor Diet and Lifestyle described in this book, I encourage you to get an endoscopic examination before you start implementing it, and again after two or three months. You will undoubtedly see dramatic changes for the better in your gastrointestinal characteristics.

In order to live a long, healthy life, do not be led astray by voices from the outside, but rather, tilt your head and listen to the voices coming from within your own body.

Chapter 2

The Enzyme Factor Diet

"You are what you eat," as the saying goes. Illnesses, life and health are the result of what you eat on a daily basis.

In 1996, influenced by the McGovern Report in the United States, Japan's Ministry of Health, Labour and Welfare decided to change the designation of what were then called "adult illnesses," such as cancer, heart disease, liver disease, diabetes, cerebral vascular disease, hypertension and hyperlipidemia (high cholesterol), to "lifestyle related illnesses." It had become clear to people through a re-examination of the relationship between food and health that these illnesses originated in lifestyle habits and not age.

However, in modern Western medicine, patients are hardly asked about their dietary history. I believe the reason that ulcerative colitis, Crohn's disease, connective tissue disease, and leukemia are called "incurable diseases of unknown cause" springs from a lack of solid information about people's dietary choices. If more research is done on the relationship between dietary history and diseases, we should be able to turn "unknown causes" into "known."

People who will undoubtedly develop lifestyle-related diseases at some point in their lives characteristically smoke cigarettes, consume alcohol every day, eat a lot of meat and hardly any fruits or vegetables, and consume dairy products such as milk, yogurt and butter, especially from an early age. The type of illness they develop will depend on their genetic predisposition and environment. For example, people who genetically have weak arterial blood vessels will develop hypertension, arteriosclerosis, or heart disease, and people with weak kidneys may develop diabetes. In women, fibroids, ovarian cysts and mammary diseases may progress into cancer, while in men, an enlarged prostate (prostatic hypertrophy) may turn into prostate cancer, and they might also develop lung cancer, colonic polyps, and arthritis. Although the type of illness depends on genetic and environmental factors, there is no mistake that people who have these lifestyle habits will develop some kind of illness.

Approximately two years after I began directly examining stomach and intestinal conditions using a scope, I began asking my patients about their dietary history. When a person receives a physical examination or medical consultation at a hospital, he or she may be asked about lifestyle habits. However, in most cases, these examinations focus only on the present, which is a pointless exercise. In order to understand why someone has become sick, it is necessary to understand that person's entire dietary history—in other words, when they eat, what they eat, and how frequently they eat it. Of course, some patients are unable to remember all the details, but as I continue to ask them patiently, I usually learn some interesting things. For example, for people who drink milk, even if all they drink is one glass of milk each day, their health results will differ depending on things like whether they started drinking milk soon after they were born or if they started drinking milk as an adult.

Looking at the dietary history of cancer patients, I usually find that they have had a diet consisting mainly of animal protein and dairy, such as meat, fish, eggs and milk. Furthermore, I have learned there is a direct correlation between when a person develops an illness and the timing and frequency with which a person consumes these things; in other words, the earlier in life and more frequently a person consumed an animal diet (especially meat and dairy products), the earlier he or she developed a disease. There are various types of cancer – cancers of the breast, colon, prostate, lung – but regardless of the type, this connection to an animal diet remains the same.

And no matter what type of cancer a person has, cancer patients' intestinal conditions are problematic without exception. I always urge people with any kind of cancer to get a colonoscopic examination because there is a good chance that they will develop a colonic polyp or colon cancer.

Among cancer patients I have examined, the results have been as expected. For women with breast cancer and men with prostate cancer, the probability of discovering an abnormality in their colon is high. As more American doctors are starting to recommend that their patients with breast, prostate and other types of cancer get colonoscopic examinations, these practices are becoming widely accepted in America. (If anyone reading this book currently has or has had cancer, I encourage you to get a colonoscopic examination as soon as possible.)

I am not saying that you will immediately develop an illness if you eat particular types of food. However, the effects of your eating habits will certainly accumulate inside your body. You cannot feel relieved just because no symptoms have appeared until now. Practice makes perfect, but if you practice bad habits day after day, year after year, you are likely to wind up perfectly ill.

Right now, we are surrounded by a wide range of different types of food. If you want to live a long and healthy life, you have to realize that you cannot choose what you eat simply because it tastes good. Knowing this, what are the criteria for choosing the foods you eat every day?

EAT FOODS THAT CONTAIN PLENTY OF ENZYMES

Since childhood, I have had a special gift of getting along immediately with any kind of dog. It is not very difficult. All you have to do is put some of your saliva in your palm and have the dog lick your hand. By doing this, you will instantly become friends with any dog.

I have raised many dogs since I was little, and I know that dogs like to lick a person's mouth. As I pondered the reason for this, I eventually realized that they like saliva. When I tested my theory, all dogs I encountered wagged their tails happily. I was only a schoolboy when I first used this method to become friends, one by one, with the neighborhood dogs. Of course at that time, I did not understand why dogs liked saliva so much. That mystery was solved when I became a doctor and began taking notice of enzymes.

"That's it! Dogs want the enzymes in saliva!"

From this, I also began to see that all animals are seeking enzymes.

When carnivorous animals such as lions capture their prey, they always first start eating the internal organs, the treasure troves of enzymes. Eskimos, who live in severely cold areas where hardly any plants grow, always eat the internal organs of their captured seal first. Rabbits eat their once-excreted stool in order to reabsorb undigested food and enzymes.

Recently, diseases in pets have suddenly increased, but you can probably guess the cause of that. The cause is pet food. Pet food is said to provide balanced nutrition, but that claim is based on modern nutrition theories, which persistently ignore enzymes. Even if the food contains enough calories and nutrients, such as vitamins, minerals, proteins and fat, if it contains no enzymes, the living thing cannot support itself. Those precious enzymes are sensitive to heat and will break down between 118.4°-239°F. Despite that, pet food is always heated during the manufacturing process regardless of whether it is canned or dry. In other words, enzymes are lost during the manufacturing process.

Wild animals do not eat food that has been heated. In the near future, I believe it will become evident that even many kinds of pet illnesses are also lifestyle-related.

The pet food problem applies to human food as well.

Currently nutritionists focus on calories and nutrients.

"Don't consume too many calories and try to eat a well-balanced nutritional meal." This is the mantra of modern dietitians.

It is commonly recommended that men consume about 2000 calories and women 1600 calories every day, and these calories are balanced across the four food groups. The first group consists of milk products and eggs — foods containing high quality protein, fat, calcium, vitamins A and B2 — the so-called "complete" nutritional foods. The second group consists of foods that build muscles and blood — products like meat, fish and legumes/beans that contain high quality protein, fats, vitamins B1 and B2 and calcium. The third group is vegetables and fruits, foods that contain vitamins, minerals and fiber and maintain the body's overall health. Finally, the fourth group consists of grains, sugars, oils and fats: foods that serve to maintain the body's temperature and energy. These foods contain carbohydrates, fats and proteins.

As you can see, the word "enzyme" is nowhere to be seen.

It is true that ascertaining the number of enzymes in food is not easy. Just as there are individual differences in the number of enzymes in each of our bodies, the number varies from food to food and even within the same food type, between each individual piece. For example, the number of enzymes found in two apples of the same variety will differ depending on each apple's environment and how many days have passed since each apple was harvested.

In the lifestyle I advocate, I basically consider foods containing many enzymes as "good food" and foods with few or no enzymes as "bad food." For that reason, the best foods are ones grown in fertile land, rich with minerals, without the use of agricultural chemicals or chemical fertilizers, and eaten immediately after being harvested.

The fresher the vegetables, fruits, meats and fishes are, the more enzymes they have. When we eat fresh food, it usually tastes good because it is packed with plenty of enzymes. However, humans differ from other animals in that we eat cooked food. We boil, bake, broil, grill, and fry food. Since enzymes are sensitive to heat, the more you cook something the more enzymes are lost. But then again, most of us cannot eat everything raw.

Therefore, it becomes very important to know how to choose the right food, how to cook it and how to eat it. Read on, and all these details will become clear.

YOUR BODY WILL BECOME OXIDIZED IF YOU CONTINUE EATING OXIDIZED FOODS

Fresh foods are considered good for the body because, aside from containing many enzymes, they are not oxidized.

Oxidation occurs when matter bonds with oxygen and "rusts." You may wonder how food, which is not metal, could rust, but we see food rusting on a daily basis.

For instance, when we fry something, the oil used becomes discolored and black. Also, apples and potatoes change color and become brown shortly after their skins are peeled. This is all attributable to oxidation, the effect of oxygen found in air. Free radicals are created when these oxidized foods enter the body.

Thanks to recent discussions of this on television shows and in magazines, you are probably already aware that free radicals are known to destroy DNA in cells, causing cancer and many other health problems. A myriad of programs focus on how to combat free radicals. It is said that red wine is good for the body because it contains the antioxidant agent polyphenol. Isoflavin, found in soybean products, is also drawing attention because it contains antioxidants as well. The reason free radicals are feared so much is because they have strong oxidation ability (the power to rust things) many times greater that that of normal oxygen.

Oxidized foods are not the only things that produce free radicals. Alcohol, tobacco and other various factors produce them as well. To begin with, free radicals are produced even by breathing. When humans breathe oxygen and burn glucose and fat in the cells that are producing energy; 2% of the oxygen taken into the body consists of free radicals.

Free radicals are often treated as the "bad guy," but in fact, they also have an essential function that enables them to kill viruses, bacteria, molds and suppress infections. However, when the numbers of free radicals increase above a certain level, the cell membranes and DNA of normal cells start to be destroyed.

When free radicals increase too much, our bodies are equipped with the means of neutralizing them—antioxidant enzymes. The type of enzyme that performs this function is called SOD (super oxide dismutase).

However, when you pass the age of 40, the amount of SOD in your body suddenly decreases. There are theories that many lifestyle-related diseases appear around the time you pass 40 because of the decrease in this enzyme.

When SODs begin to decrease with age, source enzymes start battling excess free radicals. If source enzymes are abundantly available, they focus on the free radicals as the need arises. However if source enzymes are scarce, they cannot prevent the health damage caused by the free radicals.

In short, if you continue to eat oxidized foods, it will create large numbers of free radicals in your body. Moreover, oxidized foods have very few or no enzymes at all, so the body will have difficulty producing source enzymes, leading to a vicious cycle of non-neutralized free radicals causing illnesses.

In contrast, if you eat fresh food rich with enzymes, in addition to limiting the amount of free radicals produced, you can also limit the depletion of source enzymes in your body. This will lead to a positive cycle that will steadily increase your life energy.

THERE IS NO FAT WORSE FOR YOUR BODY THAN MARGARINE

The most easily oxidized type of food is oil.

In the natural world, oils are found in the seeds of various plants. Since rice is also a "seed," there is plenty of plant oil found in brown rice. What we normally call "oil" gets squeezed from the seeds of plants. There are many types of cooking oil, such as canola oil, olive oil, sesame oil, cottonseed oil, corn oil and grape seed oil, but only the oil part is artificially extracted.

In the past, oil was usually extracted by a primitive compression process using machines, but nowadays, only a handful of manufacturers still utilize this compression process. Why? Because, not only is the process time-consuming and labor-intensive, but the loss of oil is also great. Moreover, since heat is not added at the extraction stage, the quality of the oil changes faster than that produced by other methods.

Presently, most oils generally sold on the market are produced with a chemical extraction method in which they put a chemical solvent called hexane into the raw material, heating the muddy substance. The oil is then extracted by evaporating only the solvent chemical using high pressure and heat. With this method, there is less loss of oil and, since it is heated, it is harder for the quality to change. But the oil extracted by this method becomes a trans fatty acid, or trans fat, a very destructive element for the body.

Trans fatty acids do not exist in nature and have been reported to raise the level of bad cholesterol in the body while lowering good cholesterol. They also cause cancer, hypertension and heart disease, among other health problems. In Western countries, there is a maximum level set for the number of trans fatty acids that can be found in foods, and anything exceeding that level is prohibited from being sold. In late 2006, the New York City Board of Health voted to ban trans fats at all city restaurants by July 2008.

The food that contains the most trans fatty acids is margarine. Many people believe oil extracted from vegetables, like margarine, containing no cholesterol, is better for the body than animal fats like butter. But that is a huge misconception. The truth is, *there is no type of oil worse for your body than margarine.* When I provide advice to my patients about their diet, I go so far as to say, "If you have margarine in your house, throw it away immediately."

Vegetable oils are liquids at room temperature because they contain many unsaturated fatty acids. On the other hand, animal fats, even though they are also a type of oil, are solid at room temperature because they contain many saturated fatty acids. Margarine, even though it is made with vegetable oil, is solid at room temperature, just like animal fats.

Margarine is like this because it is hydrogenated and artificially converted from unsaturated fatty acid to saturated fatty acid. In making margarine, manufacturers start with vegetable oil made by the chemical extraction method and thus containing trans fats. Hydrogen is then added, deliberately changing unsaturated fatty acids to saturated fatty acids. Thus, in margarine you have the worst of both worlds, the trans fats of chemically extracted vegetable oil and saturated fats like animal fats. There is no oil or fat worse for your body than margarine.

Shortening is another type of oil containing the same amount of trans fatty acids as margarine. I assume shortening is rarely used for cooking at home these days, but plenty of shortening is used in producing things like the cookies and snacks sold in stores and in the preparation of fast food french fries. The trans fatty acids are the reason that such sweets and fast foods are so bad for the body.

IF YOU MUST OCCASIONALLY EAT FRIED FOODS ...

How fried foods affect you depends upon where your ancestors came from, and how long "your people" have been using hot oil to cook their food. People who live in countries near the Mediterranean Sea, like Greece and Italy, have widely cultivated and used olives and olive oil for centuries, dating back nearly 6000 years. On the other hand, Japanese people began eating fried food approximately 150–200 years ago.

These differences in dietary culture may be incorporated in our genes, determining whether or not we have a digestive system that can digest oil. Oil is broken down and digested in the pancreas, but from my clinical data, it appears that the pancreas in Japanese people is weaker than the pancreas of people in countries with long histories of eating fried foods.

There are many cases of Japanese complaining about pain around their epigastric region (upper part of the stomach), but when an endoscopic examination is performed, there is no gastritis, gastric ulcers, or duodenal ulcers present. When blood tests are performed in these people, most results show an abnormally high level of amylase in the pancreas. When I ask them about their dietary history, I often find that they love to eat fried foods. However, not many Westerners who eat the same or even greater amounts of fried foods develop problems with their pancreas.

If you eat fried food two or three times a week and feel pain in the upper region of your stomach, there is a possibility that you have pancreatitis, and I would recommend that you get your pancreas examined as soon as possible.

Thinking vegetable oil is safer, people these days use it instead of animal fat. All people need to be extra careful about the amount of fried foods they eat. As I said earlier, frequent consumption of vegetable oil that has been artificially extracted is bad for the body. But if you find it impossible to stop eating fried foods, you should at least try to cut down on the number of times you eat it. The aim should be to refrain from eating fried foods more than once a month, at most.

I hardly eat fried foods myself, but when on occasion I do, I remove the batter and try as hard as possible not to consume the oily part. If you can't resist eating the outer oily parts, you should at least try to chew well. Chewing well and mixing the oily food with saliva helps neutralize trans fatty acids to a degree. Nevertheless, fried foods generally will exhaust your body's enzymes.

Moreover, oxidation occurs extremely quickly in foods cooked in oil. Since oils are not normally good for your body, you should never eat fried foods that have been sitting around for a while, like those found in many fast-food restaurants.

WHAT IS THE BEST WAY TO TAKE IN
ESSENTIAL FATTY ACIDS?

The main component of oil, fatty acids, is generally classified as either saturated fatty acids or unsaturated fatty acids. Unsaturated fatty acids are the so-called good fatty acids and are a necessary nutrient for the maintenance of the heart, circulatory organs, brain and skin. Among unsaturated fatty acids, there are some that cannot be created in the human body and therefore need to be obtained from foods. These are called essential fatty acids. They include linoleic acid, linolenic acid and arachidonic acid.

In America some years ago, people were told to take a teaspoonful of olive oil everyday to get some essential fatty acids. At the time, this was a popular practice because it was believed to be good for you. However, reports came out afterwards saying that consuming olive oil everyday could potentially cause ovarian cancer. The practice quickly died down after the report came out.

The fact is, unsaturated fatty acids have properties that cause olive oil to oxidize very easily. Even if olive oil is made from compression, I still cannot recommend consuming oil that has been artificially extracted.

If you want to consume unsaturated fatty acids, the ones found in fish are the safest bet.

There are many good quality fatty acids like DHA (Docosahexaenoic acid) and EPA (Eicosapentaenoic acid) found especially in "blue fishes," such as sardines and mackerel. Also found in the fatty part of the eyes of tuna, DHA and EPA are said to improve the functions of the brain.

It is not necessary to take oil straight if you eat foods in their natural form, since you can get the necessary unsaturated fatty acids from fats found in food. No matter what kind of oil you use, once exposed to air, it will immediately begin to oxidize. Thus, oil should not be used for cooking if at all possible.

In general, it is said that vitamin A can be absorbed better if the food is cooked with oil. Therefore, it is commonly recommended to use oil when cooking ingredients containing vitamin A. That is because vitamin A is fat-soluble and can easily be dissolved in oil.

Although it is true that vitamin A is a fat-soluble vitamin, with a little innovation it can be sufficiently absorbed without adding artificially-extracted oil because you need only a very small amount of oil to absorb fat-soluble vitamins. Thus, even if you do not use oil in the cooking process, just eating a little food that contains oil, such as soybeans and sesame seeds, will enable you to sufficiently absorb the vitamins.

In other words, you can take in a sufficient amount of oil and fats essential to the body by eating foods with fat in their natural form without adding artificially extracted oil. When I say in their natural form, I mean taking foods that are the raw material for oil, such as grains, beans, nuts and plant seeds, and eating them as they are. There is no safer or healthier way to take in oil.

MILK SOLD IN STORES IS OXIDIZED FAT

Next to oil, the most easily oxidized type of food is store-bought milk. Before being processed, milk contains many good elements. For example, it contains many types of enzymes, such as those that break down lactose; lipase, which breaks down fat; and protease, an enzyme that breaks down protein. Milk in its natural state also contains lactoferrin, known to have antioxidant, anti-inflammatory, anti-viral and immune regulatory effects.

However, milk sold in stores loses all of these good qualities through the manufacturing process. The process by which milk is manufactured is as follows. First, a suction machine is attached to the cow's nipple, squeezing out the milk, which is then stored temporarily in a tank. The raw milk collected at each farmhouse is then transferred into an even bigger tank, where it is stirred and homogenized. What actually gets homogenized are the fat droplets found in raw milk.

Raw milk consists of about 4% fat, but most of the fat consists of fat particles that exist as small droplets. Because fat particles float more easily the bigger they are, if raw milk is left alone, the fat becomes a layer of cream floating on top. When I drank bottled milk once or twice as a child, I remember seeing a layer of white creamy fat underneath the bottle caps. Since the milk was not homogenized, the fat particles had floated to the top during the transportation process.

Now, a machine called a homogenizer is used, and fat particles are mechanically broken into small pieces. The end product of this is homogenized milk. However, when homogenization occurs, the milk fat found in raw milk bonds with oxygen, changing it into hydrogenated fat (oxidized fat). Hydrogenated fat means fat that has oxidized too much, has rusted, if you will. Like all hydrogenated fat, the fat in whole homogenized milk is bad for the body.

But the manufacturing process of milk is not finished yet. Before going to market, homogenized milk must be heat-pasteurized in order to suppress the propagation of various germs and bacteria. There are four basic ways to pasteurize milk:

1. Sustained low temperature pasteurization (LTLT=low temperature long time). Pasteurization by heating at 144°–149°F for 30 minutes. This is generally called the low temperature pasteurization method.

2. Sustained high temperature pasteurization (HTLT=high temperature long time). Pasteurization by heating at over 167°F for more than 15 minutes.

3. High temperature short time method (HTST) — Pasteurization at over 161.6°F for over 15 seconds. This is the most widely used pasteurization method worldwide.

4. Ultra high temperature short time pasteurization (UHT) — Pasteurization by heating at 248–266°F for 2 seconds (or at 302°F for 1 second).

The most widely used methods in the world are the high temperature short time method and the ultra high temperature short time pasteurization process. I will repeatedly say this: Enzymes are sensitive to heat, and they begin breaking down at 118.4°F; they are completely destroyed at 239°F. Thus, irrespective of the amount of time the process takes, when the temperature reaches 266°F, *the enzymes are almost completely lost.*

Moreover, the amount of oxidized fat increases even more at ultra high temperatures, and heat changes the quality of proteins in milk. Just as the yolk of an egg that has been boiled for a long time falls apart easily, similar changes occur to proteins in milk. Lactoferrin, which is sensitive to heat, is also lost.

Because it is homogenized and pasteurized, milk sold in supermarkets throughout the world is not good for you.

COW'S MILK IS PRIMARILY FOR CALVES

Nutrients found in milk are suitable for growing calves. What is necessary for the growth of a calf is not necessarily useful for humans. Moreover, in the natural world, the only animals that drink milk are newborns. No animal drinks milk after becoming an adult (except Homo sapiens). That is how nature works. Only humans deliberately take another species' milk, oxidize it and drink it. It goes against natural law.

In Japan and the United States, children are encouraged to drink milk at school lunches because milk, which is rich in nutrients, is thought to be good for a growing child. However, anyone who thinks cow's milk and human breast milk are the same is gravely mistaken.

If you line up the various nutrients found in both cow's milk and human breast milk, they do seem very similar. Nutrients like protein, fat, lactose, iron, calcium, phosphorus, sodium, potassium and vitamins, are found in both. However, the qualities and amounts of these nutrients are completely different.

The main protein component found in cow's milk is called caseine. I have already touched upon the fact that this protein is very difficult to digest in the human gastrointestinal system. In addition, cow's milk also contains the antioxidant substance lactoferrin, which improves functions of the immune system. However, the amount of lactoferrin found in breast milk is 0.15% whereas the amount found in cow's milk is only 0.01%.

Apparently, newborns of different species require different amounts and ratios of the nutrients.

And what about adults?

Lactoferrin provides an example. Lactoferrin in cow's milk breaks down in stomach acid, so even if you drink raw milk that hasn't been heat-treated, the lactoferrin will get broken down in the stomach. This is the same for lactoferrin found in breast milk. A newborn human baby can properly absorb lactoferrin from breast milk because its stomach is underdeveloped, and since there is little stomach acid secretion, the lactoferrin does not get broken down. In other words, human breast milk is not meant to be consumed by a human adult.

Cow's milk, even if it is fresh raw milk, is not a suitable food for humans. We turn raw milk, which is not good for us to begin with, into bad food by homogenizing and pasteurizing it at high temperatures. Then, we insist our children drink it.

Another problem is that people of most ethnic groups do not have enough of the enzyme lactase to break down lactose. Most people have sufficient amounts of this enzyme when they are infants, but it decreases with age. When these people drink milk, they experience symptoms such as stomach rumblings or diarrhea, results of their bodies' inability to digest the lactose. People who completely lack lactase or have extremely few of these enzymes are called lactose intolerant. Few people are completely lactose intolerant, but some 90% of Asians; 75% of Hispanics, American Indians, and African Americans; as well as 60% of people of Mediterranean cultures and 15% of people of northern European stock lack a sufficient amount of this enzyme.

Lactose is a sugar that only exists in mammalian milk. Milk is only for newborn infants to drink. Even though many grown people lack lactase, when they are newborn infants, all healthy babies have enough for their needs. Moreover, the amount of lactose in breast milk is about 7% as opposed to 4.5% in cow's milk.

Since people, when they are babies, are able to drink breast milk rich with lactose but end up losing the enzyme as they grow up, I believe this is nature's way of saying that milk is not something a grownup should drink.

If you simply love the taste of milk, I strongly suggest you limit the frequency and try to drink milk that has not been homogenized and has been pasteurized at a low temperature. Children and adults who dislike milk should never be urged to drink it.

Drinking milk simply does not do any good for the body.

WHY TOO MUCH ANIMAL PROTEIN IS TOXIC

In the Enzyme Factor Diet and Lifestyle, I advise my patients to eat mostly grains and vegetables, and limit animal products, such as meat, fish, dairy products and eggs, keeping their intake to less than 15% of the calories consumed in any given day.

Many nutritionists currently tout animal protein as having many ideal elements, which get broken down and absorbed by amino acids in the intestine, and eventually turn into blood or muscle. However, no matter how good the food is, if you consume more than is necessary, it will become poisonous to the body. This is especially true if you consume large amounts of animal protein, because it will not be completely broken down and absorbed by the gastrointestinal system. Instead, it will decompose in the intestine, producing large amounts of toxins, such as hydrogen sulfide, indole, methane gas, ammonia, histamine and nitrosamine. In addition to these, free radicals are also produced. And in order to detoxify these toxins, large amounts of enzymes are exhausted in the intestine and liver.

The necessary amount of protein a person needs is approximately 1 gram per 1 kilogram (2.2 lbs.) of body weight. In other words, for a person whose body weight is 135 pounds, 60 grams of animal protein per day is sufficient. But in reality, there are data showing the actual protein consumption in the USA ranges from 88 to 92 grams for men and from 63 to 66 grams for women. This is obviously too much.

Proteins consumed in excess are excreted as urine in the end, but in the meantime, much harm is done to the body. First, excess proteins are converted into amino acids by digestive enzymes, and these amino acids are then broken down further in the liver before flowing into the bloodstream. Because the blood then becomes more acidic, large amounts of calcium are drawn out from bones and teeth in order to neutralize the acid. The calcium and oxidized blood are then filtered through the kidneys, with the excess protein getting excreted along with a large amount of water and calcium. Needless to say, large numbers of enzymes are consumed during this process as well.

If you ingest an excess amount of protein by consuming meat (including processed foods containing meat) and milk (including all dairy products), the damage to your health can be even more serious. Why? Because these animal foods do not contain dietary fiber, they accelerate the deterioration of your intestinal health.

Dietary fiber cannot be broken down by human digestive enzymes. Typical examples are cellulose and pectin found in plants and chitin found in the shells of crabs and shrimp.

If you eat a lot of meat and lack dietary fiber, the amount of stool decreases, causing constipation and stagnant stools. Furthermore, if this condition is left alone, diverticuli (pocket-like cavities) develop on the intestinal walls where toxins and stagnant stools have accumulated, causing polyps and cancer to develop.

WHY THE FAT IN FISH DOES NOT CLOG HUMAN ARTERIES

I have so far mentioned only meat when talking about animal protein, but even fish may pose the same health risks, if taken in excess.

According to my clinical data, however, there is one conclusive difference between meat-diet intestines" and "fish-diet intestines." That is, my patients whose diet is centered on fish do not develop diverticuli, no matter how bad their other intestinal characteristics become. In many medical books nowadays, you may read that whether it is meat, fish, or dairy products, consuming a lot of food that lacks dietary fiber will lead to diverticulosis. But from my own clinical experience, I have seen that people who eat very little or no meat but plenty of fish have spastic, rigid intestinal walls but do not go so far as to develop diverticulosis.

What causes these differences in intestinal characteristics? I believe the difference is in the type of fat found in meat versus that found in fish.

It is said the difference between the fat in meat and fish is that saturated fatty acids (meat) are bad for the body, whereas unsaturated fatty acids (fish) are good because they lower your cholesterol level. But there is an easier way to think about this, namely, by taking human as the standard. The fat of an animal whose body temperature is higher than human body temperature should be considered bad, and the fat of an animal whose body temperature is lower than human body temperature can be considered good.

The body temperature of a cow, pig or bird is normally 101.3°-104°F, higher than human body temperature (98.6°F). A chicken's body temperature is even higher at 106.7°F. The fat of these animals is in its most stable state at that particular animal's body temperature. Thus, when that fat enters the lower-temperature environment of the human body, it becomes sticky and hardens. This sticky fat thickens the blood. The flow of thickened blood is sluggish, and inside the blood vessels it becomes stagnant and clogs.

On the other hand, because fish are cold-blooded animals, under normal conditions their body temperatures are far lower than those of humans. What happens when fish fat enters the human body? Like fat you heat in a frying pan, it melts and becomes fluid. Oil in fish, as it enters the bloodstream of the human, causes the blood to become fluid, lowering the level of bad cholesterol in the blood.

Even when one consumes the same number of fat grams, fish are clearly better than warm-blooded animals for the human body because fish fat enters the bloodstream as a fluid.

THE KEY TO EATING RED MEAT FISH IS EATING IT WHILE IT IS FRESH

Fish can broadly be divided into red meat and white meat fish.

White meat fish are generally considered better for your health than red meat fish because red meat fish tend to oxidize faster. They oxidize more easily because they contain a lot of iron.

Tuna and bonito are called red meat fish because their muscular tissue is red. The red color occurs because their muscles contain special proteins called myoglobins.

Myoglobins are globular proteins that store oxygen and are formed from a chain of polypeptides, which are amino acids, and polyferrin, a type of iron. Myoglobins can be found in the muscles of animals that swim underwater for long periods of time, such as dolphins, whales and seals. This occurs because myoglobins are able to store oxygen in cells until the oxygen is needed for metabolism. Animal muscles in general are also red because of myoglobin.

Tuna and bonito have a lot of myoglobin because they swim around the ocean at tremendous speed, requiring their muscles to be continuously supplied with large amounts of oxygen. To prevent a shortage of oxygen, they have large amounts of myoglobin in their muscles. Because red meat fish contain a lot of myoglobin, they immediately oxidize once they are filleted and exposed to air. This is the reason red meat fish are considered relatively unhealthy. On the other hand, white meat fish do not contain myoglobin. Thus, even if they are cut up and filleted, they do not oxidize as quickly.

However, red meat fish have more antioxidant agents like DHA and EPA. Furthermore, an abundant amount of iron is found in myoglobin in its natural form, so it can be very good for those who are anemic. But when this iron oxidizes, it becomes ferrous oxide, which causes more harm to a body than any improvement its consumption might make in an anemic condition. Therefore, when eating red meat fish, you have to be careful to choose the freshest one.

I love tuna sushi, so when I occasionally eat it, I always have about 5mm of the surface cut out before they prepare it for me in order to remove the part that has been exposed to the air for a longer time and oxidized.

With just a little time and energy, red meat fish can be turned into a high quality food. For example, there is a local specialty in the prefecture of Kochi called *katsuo no tataki* (seared raw bonito). It involves a cooking method in which the surface of the fish is quickly seared, changing the quality of the protein and thus preventing the fish from oxidizing even when it is exposed to air. Because of the speed with which it is seared, the topmost layer of the fish protects the remainder from being exposed to ogygen, preventing oxidation from occurring. Incidentally, this cooking method also has the advantage of killing parasites that tend to gather in the skin of the fish.

Despite this, since fish is still an animal protein, you must be careful not to consume too much of it. Moreover, there have been recent reports that mercury content in tuna is on the rise. Blood tests have shown some people with tremendous elevations in the mercury level in their blood. If you are one of those people who frequently eat tuna, please get yourself examined at least once. We all need to recognize that ground and sea pollution are directly connected to our individual health, so we must be careful in this regard.

AN IDEAL MEAL CONSISTS OF 85% FROM
PLANTS AND 15% FROM ANIMALS

The Enzyme Factor Diet and Lifestyle advises that the ratio of fruits, vegetables, legumes and grains to meat in our diet be 85% to 15% respectively. I am frequently asked, "If I decrease meat in my diet by so much, won't I lack essential proteins?" I tell people who ask this question not to worry. Even with a vegan diet, one can get enough protein.

Like most animals and plants, the human body is mainly built from proteins. But even if you eat a lot of food with protein, like meat and fish, it does not necessarily mean that protein will be used directly to build up your body. That is because proteins are formed from amino acids, and amino acids vary in their arrangements.

In the human intestine, proteins get absorbed by the intestinal walls only after being broken down by digestive enzymes into amino acids. The absorbed amino acids then get resynthesized in the body into the necessary proteins.

There are approximately 20 kinds of amino acids forming human proteins. Of the 20, eight cannot be synthesized by the human body. Those eight amino acids are lysine, methionine, tryptophan, valine, threonine, leucine, isoleucine and phenylalanine, collectively called "essential amino acids." These amino acids are precious because if you lack even one of them, there is a possibility of serious nutritional disorder. That is why it is absolutely necessary to include them in your diet every day.

Animal proteins are considered good quality proteins since they contain all of the essential amino acids. It is because of this that modern nutritionists tell you to have animal proteins every day. But plant proteins also contain many, although not all, of the essential amino acids. Grains, cereals, legumes, vegetables, mushrooms, fruits and sea vegetables all contain many amino acids. Many people are surprised when they are told that 37% of *nori* (dried seaweed) is protein, but many people know that the sea vegetable kelp is a treasure house of amino acids.

Among all vegetable foods, soybeans are considered the "meat of the fields" because they contain an abundance of amino acids. The amount of essential amino acids in soybeans, except for the slightly-less-than-standard levels of threonine, is hardly inferior compared to meat, and they will digest much more easily, without depleting your source enzymes as meat does.

Of course, consuming too much plant protein is not good, but if you consider the fact that plants contain a lot of dietary fiber and no animal fat, I would recommend that you center your diet on plant proteins, supplementing them occasionally with a little animal protein, preferably fish.

If you look at the various plant foods individually, it is true that no single vegetable has all of the essential amino acids. But we normally do not eat just one type of food in any meal. If you skillfully combine grains as the staple food, main vegetables, side vegetables and soup, you can get enough essential amino acids with just a plant-based diet.

WHITE RICE IS "DEAD FOOD"

Recently, many people have started reducing their rice intake because they believe carbohydrates will make them gain weight. However, it is a mistake to think rice will make you gain weight. 40-50% of my entire diet consists of grains, but because my meals are well balanced, I never gain weight.

My staple food, however, is not the polished white rice people normally eat. It is brown rice, to which I add about five other grains, such as rolled barley, millet, buckwheat, quinoa, amaranth, oatmeal, whole oats, and bulgar. I mix these other grains with brown rice and have this as my staple food. I choose unrefined fresh whole grains, all organically grown.

The harvesting season for rice is limited, so it is not possible always to have freshly harvested rice. That is why I purchase brown rice in vacuum-packed bags to prevent the rice from being exposed to oxygen. Once that seal is broken, I try to eat it all within 10 days because rice oxidizes when exposed to air. Oxidation occurs much faster in white rice than in brown rice because the skin of white rice is hulled. It is the same thing as when peeled apples immediately change color and become brown.

The rice we eat is a seed of the rice plant. This seed is wrapped in a rice husk shell in its original state. When the rice husk is removed, we are left with what is commonly called brown rice. When all the rice bran layers have been removed, what remains is the rice germ. When this rice germ is removed, albumen, which is white rice, is the only thing left.

Most people prefer to eat white rice because it is white, soft, sweet in flavor, and looks better, but in reality, white rice is rice whose most important parts have been removed. It is dead food.

If you leave a peeled apple or potato out, it oxidizes and becomes brown. Even refined rice (although the color does not change) oxidizes much faster than brown rice since its shell has been hulled. White rice tastes really good if it is fresh from a refining machine because it has not oxidized yet.

However, white rice no longer contains the bran or germ part of the rice, so even if it is soaked in water, it will only swell up without germinating or sprouting. Brown rice, on the other hand, can sprout if soaked in water at the right temperature. It is living food, with the potential to sprout life. This is why I say that white rice is non-living, or dead, food.

Plant seeds contain many enzymes so that the plant can germinate when placed in a suitable environment. The seeds also possess a substance called trypsin inhibitors, which prevents the seed from germinating on its own. The reason it is harmful to eat grains, beans, and potatoes raw is that a large number of digestive enzymes are needed to neutralize and digest trypsin inhibitors. However, since trypsin inhibitors are broken down and become easier to digest when heat is added, it is better to eat grains, beans, and potatoes after they have been cooked

Unrefined grains are jam-packed with nutrients that are good for the body. They contain balanced amounts of important nutrients, like proteins, carbohydrates, fats, dietary fibers, vitamin B1, vitamin E and minerals such as iron and phosphorus.

No matter how good the quality of the white rice, it only has about 1/4 of the nutrients of brown rice. Many nutrients are packed in the germ part, so in eating refined rice, it is better to at least keep the germ part intact.

Many people say it is very hard to cook brown rice, but there are rice cookers on the market today that can easily handle this job. You can also get what is called *hatsuga* brown rice, which is brown rice that has germinated only slightly. Hatsuga brown rice can be cooked deliciously even in rice cookers that cannot handle cooking brown rice.

Wheat is also good as an unrefined grain. If wheat gets refined, its nutritional value will dramatically decrease. If you enjoy eating bread and pasta, it is best to choose those made of whole wheat flour.

WHY CARNIVORES EAT HERBIVORES

The basic rule of food is to eat things fresh.

Fresh things are better because the fresher the food, the more enzymes they contain. These enzymes can later be transformed into some of the 3,000 enzymes the body needs to function.

There are countless species of animals on earth, and they all have unique diets, but the one thing they all have in common is their fondness for foods rich in enzymes. Have we humans forgotten this basic rule of nature? Humans have established modern nutritional theories by examining the nutrients found in food, classifying them and counting the calories. However, the most fundamental factor, the enzyme factor, has been completely omitted. Thus, people eat a lot of dead food that contains no enzymes.

The same thing can be said of pet food. Pet food nowadays contains no enzymes. As a result, many pets suffer from various illnesses. That is why I do not give my dogs pet food. Instead, I feed them brown rice that I myself eat. It may seem strange for dogs to eat brown rice, but they are very happy when I feed them brown rice sprinkled with some *non* (seaweed). They also enjoy eating vegetables and fruits. They even fight over and devour lightly boiled broccoli stems.

When we talk about carnivores, you may think they require only meat, but that is not true. They also need vegetables. So why do they eat only meat? Because they do not have the enzymes to break down plants. But this does not mean that they lack access to exterior sources of enzymes.

You will understand this when you observe that carnivores in the wild eat only herbivores. After they capture their herbivore prey, the first things they eat are the intestines, in which the plants that were eaten by the herbivore, along with some enzymes, were in the process of being digested. In this way, the carnivore acquires the plants that were digested and in the process of being digested in the herbivore's stomach and intestines.

Carnivores eat only herbivores, and herbivores eat only plants. That is the law of nature. If you ignore this law, you will certainly suffer some repercussions. A typical example of this is BSE, or Mad Cow Disease.

The cause of BSE is not completely known at this time, but what we do know is that the brain starts turning into sponge owing to an abnormal change in prions, a protein particle that lacks nucleic acid. So what causes the abnormal change in prions? It is evident from research up to now that BSE has spread from the distribution of food containing powdered meat bones (which is feed manufactured from meat, skin and bones left over from the processing of meat). Government agencies in the United States and Japan, as well as other countries, have said BSE is due to genetically contaminated powdered meat bones. But if you ask me, giving herbivorous cows powdered meat bones in the first place goes against the laws of nature.

The practice of giving cows powdered meat bones arose from humans' narrow self-interest. Feed consisting of powdered meat bones increases the amount of protein and calcium in cow milk. Milk containing more protein and calcium can be sold at a higher price. Thus, I believe BSE is caused by the selfishness and arrogance of humans who have ignored the laws of nature.

In the end, the type and amount of food all animals, including humans, should eat is determined by the laws of nature. You cannot live a healthy life by ignoring this.

WHY HUMANS HAVE 32 TEETH

As I explained earlier, the ideal balanced meal consists of 85% plant and 15% animal foods. I came up with this ratio, in fact, from looking at the number of human teeth. Teeth reflect what type of food every species of animal should eat. For example, the teeth of carnivores are all very sharp, like canine teeth. These are well-suited for ripping the meat off the bones of their prey. In contrast, herbivores have teeth like incisor teeth, thin and square and suited for biting off plants. They also have molars, which grind up the plants once they are bitten off.

It may sound crazy to count an animal's teeth in order to judge what is the most suitable diet for that animal, but this is actually not such a novel idea. Many in the past have also asserted that there is a deep connection between types of teeth and an ideal diet.

Humans have a total of 32 teeth (including wisdom teeth). The breakdown is as follows: 2 pair of incisors (front teeth) on the top and bottom, 1 pair of canine top and bottom and 5 pair of molars on the top and bottom. Thus, in humans, the ratio is 1 canine to 2 incisors to 5 molars: 1 canine to eat meat and 2 incisors plus 5 molars totaling 7 to eat plant-based foods.

If we apply this balance between plants and meats, it comes out to a 7-to-1 ratio, and thus the ratio I suggest of a diet of 85% plant-based foods and 15% animal-based foods.

If we summarize the most balanced diet suitable for humans:

- The ratio of plant-based to animal-based food is 85–90% to 10–15% respectively.
- On the whole, grains should be 50%, vegetables and fruits 35-40%, and meat 10–15%.
- Eat unrefined grains, which on the whole constitute 50% of the diet.

You may think the vegetable portion is disproportionately large, but take a look at chimpanzees, the animal whose genes most closely resemble human genes (98.7% the same). The diet of chimpanzees is 95.6% vegetarian. The breakdown is 50% fruits, 45.6% nuts, potatoes, roots, and the remaining 4.5% is animal diet consisting mainly of insects, such as ants. They do not even eat fish.

I have examined the gastrointestines of chimpanzees with an endoscope, but they are so similar to those of humans that I could not tell just by looking whether it was that of a human or a chimp. And what surprised me most was how clean their gastrointestinal characteristics and features were.

Wild animals, unlike humans, die immediately if they become sick. They instinctively know that food is what supports their life and protects their health.

I believe that it is necessary for us humans to learn from nature and, with greater humility, return to the basic fundamentals of food.

WHY CHEWING WELL AND MODERATION ARE GOOD FOR HEALTH

In Chapter 1, I discussed how regular food that is chewed well is better for digestion than porridge, which is usually not chewed as well. But there are many other benefits to chewing well, the biggest one being the conservation of source enzymes.

I always try to chew each mouthful of food 30-50 times. If I'm chewing regular food, it turns completely mushy and goes down my throat without much effort. But when eating hard food or foods that do not digest well, I chew about 70-75 times. The human body is built in such a way that the salivary glands secrete more saliva the more one chews, and as that gets mixed well with stomach acid and bile, the digestive process proceeds smoothly.

The intestinal wall of a person can absorb substances up to 15 microns (.015 millimeter) in size, and anything bigger than that will be excreted. Thus if you do not chew well, most of the food you eat will go to waste without being absorbed.

When I tell people this, young women often say, If it doesn't get absorbed I won't gain weight, so isn't that good?" But the situation is not that simple. Decomposition and abnormal fermentation occur inside the intestine when foods are not digested and absorbed, just as in the case of excess consumption. Decomposition gives rise to various toxins, which exhaust large amounts of enzymes.

Furthermore, because there is a wide gap between the rates of absorption of easily digestible things and things that are difficult to digest, even if you eat a well-balanced meal, you can still end up lacking certain nutrients. There is especially the danger of missing nutrients that exist in trace amounts.

Recently, there has been a rise in the number of people who gain weight owing to excess intake of calories but still lack essential nutrients. This is usually caused by a badly balanced diet together with indigestion and non-absorption caused by not chewing well.

Chewing well is actually better for those who want to lose weight because it takes that much longer to eat meals. While eating, your blood sugar level rises and your appetite gets restrained, preventing you from overeating. By chewing well, you get the feeling of fullness more quickly. Thus, you do not have to muster a lot of will power and force yourself to decrease the amount you eat; you just naturally want to eat less.

Another benefit of chewing well is that it kills parasites. Nowadays, we do not see insects on vegetables, but there are still many parasites in bonito, squid, and freshwater fish. They are extremely small in size, and if not chewed well, they will be swallowed as they are and start living off of your internal organs. However, it is known that if you chew 50-70 times, the parasites can be killed inside your mouth.

Once you start choosing good ingredients for your meals, you will naturally begin to choose organic vegetables and wild fish instead of farm fish. These foods may have many insects since they are grown naturally, but you should not be afraid of parasites and insects if you know that chewing well will protect you from any potential harm.

Some people may think that the more you chew, the more saliva will be secreted in your mouth, using up more of your enzymes. But that is not the case. The number of enzymes exhausted by chewing well is much lower than the number that would be used if food that is not chewed well enters the stomach for digestion. And by chewing well, your appetite is naturally suppressed. When the amount of food you eat decreases, the number of enzymes used for digestion and absorption also decreases. So if you look at it from a whole body perspective, chewing well leads to enzyme conservation.

What this means is that source enzymes do not get used up in the digestion process so that there are more enzymes that can be used for maintaining the body's homeostasis, detoxification, repair and supply of energy. As a result, your body's resistance and immune system improve, leading to a longer life.

Moreover, if you do not overeat, most of the food will get digested and absorbed completely, and thus, there will be less chance of unabsorbed food decaying and toxins forming in the intestines. Enzymes used for detoxification will also be conserved. The fact is, if you follow the Enzyme Factor Diet and Lifestyle, your stomach and intestinal characteristics will improve in about six months, and some of the unpleasant odor of gas and stool will be alleviated.

No matter how good the food or how indispensable the nutrient, excess intake will cause harm to one's health. The important thing is to eat a well-balanced diet consisting of natural, fresh foods and to chew well. If you bear in mind these three things, you will save your source enzymes and enjoy a long life with a healthy body.

YOU CANNOT STAY HEALTHY BY EATING FOOD THAT TASTES AWFUL

In this chapter, I have talked about good foods that help sustain life and bad foods harmful to your health. The key differences between "good food" and "bad food" are enzymes and freshness. I have also discussed eating good food in the right balance and how to eat that food.

Through the process of evolution, humans have learned to cook food. We have learned to enjoy and preserve different kinds of foods as well. On the other hand, we are also losing precious enzymes by cooking our food.

In the wild, no animals eat cooked food. Moreover, they do not eat refined or processed foods. Thus, there are some researchers of diet and health who advocate completely abandoning processed foods and only eating foods in their raw state.

However, I do not believe that is the right approach. In order for a person to live a healthy life, it is important for that person to experience a sense of pleasure and wellbeing. For humans, food is a source of great pleasure. You cannot be healthy if you force yourself to eat foods that taste bad.

Therefore, the Enzyme Factor Diet and Lifestyle considers both the enjoyment of food and adherence to proper diet as important factors for maintaining one's health. To reiterate the main points of my dietary lifestyle:

- Maintain a ratio of 85-90% plant-based foods and 10–15% animal-based foods.

- Grains should constitute 50%, vegetables and fruits 35–40%, and animal foods 10–15% of the whole.

- Eat unrefined grains, which on the whole constitute 50% of the diet.

- The animal foods portion should be from animals, like fish, with a lower body temperature than humans.

- Eat fresh and unrefined foods, if possible, in their natural form.

- Avoid milk and dairy products as much as possible (people who are lactose intolerant, predisposed to allergies, or dislike milk and dairy products should completely avoid them).

- Avoid margarine and fried foods.

- Chew well (40–70 times each bite) and try to eat small meals.

It is not very difficult to continue enjoying your meals if you understand the human body's mechanism and the laws of nature, and follow these key points. The easiest way is to make this a habit from childhood.

If you find joy in eating, it is all right to eat a thick steak or cheese and drink alcohol once in awhile. If you let loose 5% of the time and are careful about what you eat the other 95% of the time, source enzymes will continue to protect your health, for health is the accumulation of long-term habits.

What is important is to follow a healthy and lasting lifestyle *that you can enjoy.*

Chapter 3

Habits of the Rich and Healthy

There is always a reason people become sick. Their eating habits are in disorder, their way of eating is wrong, their lifestyle is a mess, or all of the above.

In America since 1990, there has been a steady decline in the rates of cancer and deaths resulting from cancer. I believe this has occurred because after the McGovern Report was presented in 1977, the U.S. government began touting appropriate dietary guidelines that gradually began to penetrate American society.

In America today, the higher a person is on the socioeconomic ladder, the more serious they are about improving their eating habits. The eating habits of Americans with economic power, the so-called "upper class," are very healthy nowadays. They are eating more fruits and vegetables, and fewer fat-dripping steaks are seen on their dinner tables. Thus, there are fewer overweight people among this social class, even as obesity in America generally has reached epidemic proportions. It is said that in America, an obese person cannot become president of a company. This is because many believe that a person who cannot even manage his or her own health cannot possibly manage a company's business.

So why is there a gap in the eating habits between the upper socioeconomic class and everyone else?

One problem is the cost. Buying foods that are fresher, such as vegetables and fruits, and organic foods that were not grown with agricultural chemicals or chemical fertilizers can be very costly. It is usually the case that the better the food, the higher the price. As a result, in America today, you have the separation of the healthy, wealthy class and the unhealthy majority. I believe this trend will not be reversed, as the eating habits of each social class get passed down from parent to child within that social class.

THE MAJORITY OF DISEASES ARE CAUSED
BY HABIT, RATHER THAN HEREDITY

There are many people who, when they become middle-aged or elderly, develop the same illnesses as their parents, such as diabetes, hypertension, heart disease and cancer. When that happens, some people say, "It was inevitable I would get cancer because cancer runs in our family." But that is not so. I will not say there are no genetic factors involved, but a big cause of hereditary disease is inheriting the habits that cause the disease.

Household habits are ingrained subconsciously in children's minds as they grow up. Preferences for certain foods, cooking methods, lifestyles, and values all vary from family to family, but parents and children growing up in the same household share similar preferences. In other words, children are more prone to develop the same illnesses as their parents, not because they inherited the genes that cause the disease, but rather because they inherit lifestyle habits that cause the disease.

If children inherit good habits, such as choosing fresh ingredients and good water, living a proper lifestyle and not taking many medications, they will find it easier to maintain their health. However, by inheriting bad habits, such as eating a lot of oxidized foods, relying too much on medications, and pursuing an improper lifestyle, the children will likely become unhealthy, possibly even more so than their parents

In this way, children inherit the good or bad habits of their parents. Adults who were told by their parents from a young age that they should drink milk every day since it is good for the body are probably still drinking milk—with their parents' words ingrained in their minds. Only by reflecting carefully on our own habits, testing them against the best current nutritional information and taking responsibility can we pass down better health to the next generation.

HABITS REWRITE GENES

The older one gets, the harder it becomes to change one's habits. Moreover, habits that get imprinted in our minds while we are young often exercise a powerful influence over our entire lives. Therefore, it is important to imprint good habits on children as early as possible.

There has been substantial research and an inordinate focus placed on infant education, development of the brain, and honing concentration skills for children who are too young even to remember things. But when looking at people's awareness of health issues, there is not enough research being done. Intellectual development is an important issue for good education and social purposes, but accurate knowledge of how health habits are imprinted in children's minds is just as important. Even if you send your kids to the best schools, they cannot lead rich lives if their bodies are not healthy.

Most Americans entrust their meals to their favorite restaurants or fast-food places and their health to their doctors and know very little about the medications they are taking. If I may say so as a physician, too many people have far too little knowledge of medicine. I believe a person's physical condition is chiefly determined by the following two factors: what you inherit from your parents and the lifestyle habits you grow up with.

For example, if your parents lack sufficient enzymes to break down alcohol, you will also lack the same enzymes. However, if you gradually increase the amount of alcohol you drink, the number of enzymes used by your liver also increases and eventually you will be able to drink a fair amount of alcohol. In essence, you are building up your tolerance for alcohol

This is especially true if your parents, who did not have sufficient enzymes to break down alcohol, eventually built up a tolerance. People with such parents are likely to believe they, too, can build up tolerance if they continue drinking. On the other hand, if you see your parents who have no tolerance for alcohol refrain from drinking, then you are more likely to accept the fact that you, too, are unable to drink.

This may not be the best example, but the truth is, good habits will overcome bad genes.

Even though your parents may have had genes for cancer, if you take good care of your health, practice sensible lifestyle habits and live out your natural lifespan, your children will probably learn that genes for cancer do not necessarily have to lead to cancer, and they can follow your lead to prevent cancer from developing. In this way, as good dietary and lifestyle habits are passed down from generation to generation, "cancer genes" will steadily weaken from one generation to the next. In other words, inheriting good habits means you can "rewrite" genes.

Nor are children who were raised on bottled milk doomed to bad health in their adult years. Children who are bottle-fed because their mothers cannot breastfeed them develop allergies more easily than breastfed children. However, after being weaned off the bottled milk, if they are careful with their diet and continue to accumulate good lifestyle habits, they will not develop lifestyle-related diseases as they get older.

On the other hand, if children who were raised to be healthy by being breastfed later adopt bad habits, such as eating a lot of meat and dairy products and oxidized foods with additives, they will become susceptible to health problems.

You are born with certain hereditary factors, but habits can be changed with the power of effort. Depending on the accumulation of habits, hereditary factors can change into either a positive or a negative thing. The good habits that save you can also save the next generation.

THE WORST LIFESTYLE HABITS ARE ALCOHOL AND TOBACCO

Doctors still depend heavily on surgical operations and drugs, and it appears that not many try to raise their patients' awareness of proper dietary habits, despite widespread acknowledgment that cancer, heart disease, diabetes and many other diseases are largely related to diet.

However, even if your diet improves markedly, that alone cannot completely prevent you from developing some diseases because, aside from your diet, there are many other factors in your life that can exhaust source enzymes. In addition to a proper diet, you will also want to consciously eliminate other bad habits in order to protect your health.

The worst of those bad habits are alcohol and tobacco. The biggest reason these two are considered the worst is that they are addictive, and many people cannot go a day without drinking or smoking.

I can immediately tell whether a person is a smoker just by looking at his face. A person who smokes has a peculiar gray skin color. Your skin becomes gray when you smoke because, in addition to the capillaries constricting and preventing oxygen and nutrients from being supplied to the cells, waste and decay cannot be excreted. In other words, that graying is due to toxins accumulating in the skin cells.

When talking about the harmfulness of cigarettes, the focus is usually only on tar accumulating in the lungs. But equally serious and harmful for the body is the constriction of capillaries throughout the body. When capillaries constrict, fluids cannot flow throughout the body. If the fluids cannot flow, nutrients carried in the fluids also do not reach some parts of the body. Moreover, waste, which should be excreted, does not leave the body either. As a result, waste collects and decays, giving rise to toxins. The "blackness" appearing on the skin is easy to see, but in actuality, the same things are occurring within the body, especially in parts connected to the tips of capillaries.

The blood vessels of a person who drinks alcohol often constrict in the same way as they do in someone who smokes every day. There are those who say a small amount of alcohol opens up blood vessels, improving the circulation of the blood, but depending on the alcohol, the blood vessel can only open up for about 2-3 hours. The truth is, this "opening up of blood vessels" ultimately causes blood vessels to constrict. When you drink, your blood vessels suddenly expand. But in reaction to that, your body tries to counter by constricting them. When your blood vessels constrict, nutritious food and waste cannot be absorbed or excreted, leading to the same problems caused by smoking cigarettes.

In this way, alcohol and tobacco give rise to large numbers of free radicals inside the body. And what neutralizes them are the antioxidant agent SOD and antioxidant enzymes such as catalase, glutathione and peroxidase. It is commonly known that if you smoke frequently, large amounts of vitamin C get destroyed. That is because vitamin C is one of the antioxidant agents.

In order to neutralize free radicals, large amounts of antioxidant enzymes are used. Even though free radicals are also generated by factors in our daily lives that are beyond our control— like electromagnetic waves and environmental pollution—people also still intentionally consume things like tobacco and alcohol that are within their control. If large numbers of free radicals are produced, it means your precious source enzymes are also being consumed.

Enzymes will run out if you continue to use them rapidly, just as you will run deeply into debt very quickly if you continue to use your credit card and never pay down on it. Pursuing a good diet and practicing good habits are the same as steadily saving money. But if you keep spending large amounts of money daily, you will accumulate a daunting debt. Eventually the creditors catch up with you, and in the case of enzymes, that means you get sick. If you continue to spend without getting rid of your debt, you will go broke. In terms of your health, this bankruptcy is more serious than financial bankruptcy. It results in death.

HABITS THAT CAN CURE SLEEP APNEA SYNDROME

Many people's daily habits cause illnesses. Yet some illnesses can be cured if daily habits are slightly altered. One example of the latter is sleep apnea, a syndrome that has lately attracted much attention.

Sleep apnea syndrome is a disease in which breathing ceases intermittently during sleep. Because muscles relax during sleep, when a person sleeps lying face up, the base of that person's tongue droops down, narrowing the respiratory tract. People with sleep apnea have severe respiratory tract stricture, and because their respiratory tract closes up temporarily, breathing stops. They feel as though they are suffocating when their breathing stops, so they wake up many times during the night. Being sleep-deprived in this way, they become overwhelmingly sleepy or are unable to concentrate during the day.

This disorder will not lead to death by suffocation during sleep. However, in addition to lowering immune and metabolic functions, lack of sleep puts a burden on the circulatory system, increasing the probability of heart disease or stroke by three to four times, making this a frightening disease.

Seventy to eighty percent of patients with this disease are obese. In the beginning, it was thought that obesity caused sleep apnea by narrowing the respiratory tract, but further research has shown no such direct connection.

There are three classifications of sleep apnea. "Obstructive apnea" occurs when the respiratory tract becomes obstructed; "central apnea" occurs when the activity of the brain's respiratory center declines; and "mixed apnea"— is a mixture of the first two types. In fact, there is an easy cure to "obstructive sleep apnea," which is the most common of the three. The cure is to avoid putting anything in the stomach four or five hours before going to bed. Simply put, to cure sleep apnea, go to sleep on an empty stomach.

The human trachea is organized in such a way that nothing other than air can get in. However, if food is in the stomach before going to sleep, those contents will rise up from the stomach to the throat when you lie down. When this happens, the body narrows the respiratory tract and stops your breathing in order to prevent the contents from entering the trachea.

The fact that most people with sleep apnea syndrome are obese coincides with my hypothesis. This is because, if you eat right before going to sleep at night, large amounts of insulin get secreted. But whether you eat carbohydrates or proteins, insulin changes everything to fat. Thus, it is much easier to gain weight if you eat late at night, even if you aren't eating anything "fattening." In other words, you do not develop sleep apnea syndrome because you are obese, but rather, the habit of eating right before going to bed causes both sleep apnea syndrome and obesity.

Eating right before going to sleep at night is indeed a bad habit.

There are some drinkers who have "night caps" out of habit, thinking it is better than taking sleeping pills, but this is also dangerous. The person may feel this makes him fall asleep more easily, but the fact is, his breathing is more likely to stop intermittently, resulting in a decline in the blood oxygen level. This causes an oxygen shortage in the heart muscle, and for people with arteriosclerosis or narrowed coronary arteries, this condition can lead to death.

The cause of many people dying at daybreak from a heart attack or myocardial infarction is in fact acid reflux that occurs as a result of eating and drinking late at night, and leads in turn to the closing of the respiratory tract, irregular breathing, decrease in blood oxygen level and, finally, oxygen shortage to the heart muscle.

This risk increases if alcohol is consumed along with eating before going to sleep because, when one drinks alcohol, the respiratory center gets repressed, further decreasing the blood oxygen level. For people who have few enzymes to break down alcohol, the alcohol remains in their blood for a longer period of time, so they need to be extra careful.

Moreover, there are people who give hot milk to their children at bedtime because it helps them sleep well, but this is also a bad idea. Even if children eat dinner around 6 p.m., they will still have food in their stomachs when they go to sleep since they go to bed earlier than adults. If, on top of that, you also make them drink milk, it becomes easier for reflux to occur. As a result, breathing becomes irregular, sometimes even stopping for a moment, and when the child takes a deep breath, he or she inhales milk, which can easily become an allergen. In fact, I believe this is one of the causes of childhood asthma.

Although this has yet to be proven, according to research data I have collected from my patients, I have found that many people who had childhood asthma were sent to bed immediately after eating or being given milk at bedtime when they were young.

In order to prevent such maladies as childhood asthma, sleep apnea syndrome, myocardial infarction and heart attacks, simply make a habit of going to sleep on an empty stomach.

If, however, you simply cannot endure hunger pangs at night, eating a little fresh fruit containing plenty of enzymes about an hour before bedtime is the preferred choice. Enzymes found in fruit are extremely digestible and move from the stomach to the intestines in about 30-40 minutes. Therefore, you do not have to worry about reflux occurring after you lie down, as long as bedtime is about an hour after eating the fruit.

Drink Water One Hour Before Meals

One "good habit" I practice every day is drinking about 500cc of water one hour before all my meals.

People often say you should drink plenty of good water every day for your health, but just as there is a good time to eat meals, there is also a good time to drink water. I am sure people who grow their own plants will understand this. After all, excessive watering of plants will cause the roots to rot, and the plants will wither and die. Just as there is an appropriate time period and amount to water plants, the same can be said of regarding human consumption of water.

The human body is made mostly of water. Babies and small children are composed of approximately 80% water, adults 60-70% and the elderly 50-60%. Babies have fresh and youthful looking skin because their cells contain a lot of water. It is very important for the human body to be supplied with plenty of fresh, good water.

Water that enters the mouth gets absorbed by the gastrointestinal system before being transported to cells throughout the body via blood vessels. More water makes the blood flow better, promoting efficient metabolism. Good water also has the effect of decreasing the level of cholesterol and triglycerides in the blood. Thus, adults should drink at least 6-8 cups of water every day, and the elderly should drink at least 5 cups.

When is the right time to drink water?

If you consume too much water right before meals, your stomach will become full, causing you to lose your appetite. And, if you drink water during meals, it will dilute the digestive enzymes in your stomach, making it more difficult to digest and absorb the food. Thus, if you need to drink water during your meals, you should avoid drinking more than a cup during each meal.

Still, there are doctors who advise people to drink water before going to bed or when they wake up during the night—even if they are not thirsty—in order to prevent their blood from thickening. However, I oppose this practice. You should avoid drinking water before going to bed if you want to prevent reflux from occurring. Even if it is only water, when water mixes with stomach acid, enters the trachea and is inhaled into the lungs, you run the chance of getting pneumonia.

The ideal way to supply your body is to drink water after waking up in the morning and one hour before each meal. If it is only water, it will move from the stomach to the intestine in 30 minutes and, consequently, it will not hinder digestion or absorption.

This is my daily routine for drinking water:

• Drink 1–3 cups first thing in the morning

• Drink 2–3 cups one hour before lunch

• Drink 2–3 cups one hour before dinner

Of course, this is only one way to do it. During the summer, everyone needs more water, especially those who sweat heavily. However, people with weak gastrointestinal systems may end up with diarrhea if they drink too much water. The amount of water a person needs differs depending on that person's body size and needs to be determined by what is deemed appropriate for that individual's body. If drinking 6 cups of water causes diarrhea, then decrease the amount you drink to 1.5 cups three times a day, gradually increasing the amount over time.

During cold weather, heat water slightly and then drink it slowly. Drinking cold water will cool the body. It is said the body temperature at which enzymes become the most active is around 96.8–104°F. Moreover, if the body temperature rises 1°F within this limit, it is said that the immune system increases its effectiveness by 35%. I believe fevers occur during illnesses as a part of the body's natural defenses, because the rise in body temperature activates these enzymes.

WATER AND SOURCE ENZYMES ARE GOOD PARTNERS

Water has many functions inside the human body, but the biggest function is to improve blood flow and promote metabolism. It also activates the intestinal bacterial flora and enzymes while excreting waste and toxins. Dioxins, pollutants, food additives and carcinogens are all flushed out of the body by good water.

For all these reasons, people who do not drink enough water will get sick more easily.

Conversely, if you drink plenty of good water, it will be harder for you to get sick. When water moistens areas of the body where bacteria and viruses can invade most easily, such as the bronchi and gastrointestinal mucosa, the immune system is activated, making those areas difficult for viruses to invade.

In contrast, if not enough water is consumed, the bronchial mucous membranes dehydrate and dry out. Phlegm and mucus are produced in the bronchus (*i.e.,* the bronchial tube), but if there is not enough water, they will stick to the bronchus, making it a breeding ground for bacteria and viruses.

Water is not only present inside the blood vessels but also plays an active role inside lymph vessels, thus helping us maintain our health. If blood vessels are like a river, the lymph vessel system of the human body is like a sewage pipe. It carries out the important functions of purifying, filtering, and transporting excess water, proteins, and waste through the bloodstream. Inside the lymph vessels are antibodies called gamma globulins, which have immune functions and enzymes called lysozymes that have antibacterial effects. In order for the immune system to function properly, good water is absolutely necessary.

Water is vital to all parts of the body. A body cannot sustain itself without adequate water. That is the reason why plants do not grow in the desert. In order for plants to grow, sunlight, soil and water are all you need. If you have only sunlight and dirt, nutrients cannot be absorbed; thus the plant will wither and die. Water makes it possible for nutrients to be absorbed by the plant.

In a human being, if water is not distributed properly, that person will not only become malnourished, but waste and toxins will also accumulate inside the cells, unable to be excreted. In the worst-case scenario, the accumulated toxins will damage cell genes, causing some cells to become cancerous.

Whether to improve the flow of the gastrointestinal system or the flow of blood and lymph fluids, water has very broad functions in the body.

Providing nourishment to and receiving and disposing of waste from the body's 60 trillion cells are microfunctions of water. These microfunctions, which produce energy and break down free radicals, also involve many enzymes.

In other words, if water is not precisely distributed to all 60 trillion cells, enzymes will not be able sufficiently to accomplish those functions. In order for enzymes to work properly, not only are various trace nutrients such as vitamins and minerals needed, but they also require the medium in which these things are transported, namely, water.

Moreover, the amount of water a person excretes in a day, including sweat that evaporates, is said to be approximately 10.5 cups. Of course there is water in food, but even when you consider that, it is necessary to replenish at least six or seven cups of water per day.

When I tell people to drink plenty of fluids, some say, "I do not drink a lot of water, but I do drink plenty of tea and coffee." For the human body, though, it is very important to get water. When we consume fluids other than water, such as tea, coffee, carbonated drinks and beer, instead of supplementing the fluids in the body, these fluids actually cause dehydration. Sugar, caffeine, alcohol and additives contained in these drinks rob fluids from the body's cells and blood, making the body's blood thicker.

Many people chug a mug of beer on a hot summer day or after coming out of a sauna. Although beer may be refreshing when you are very thirsty, middle-aged and elderly people with high cholesterol, high blood pressure or diabetes are more likely to experience myocardial infarction, (heart attack) or brain infarction (stroke) if they rely on beer to replace the water lost through sweating.

If you get thirsty, instead of drinking beer, tea, or coffee, make it a habit to first drink good water, firmly supplying your body with the fluid it needs.

"Good Water" Is Water with Strong Deoxidation Qualities

I trust that you now understand just how important it is to drink good water. But you may want to ask what kind of water can be considered good water?

When I say "good water," I doubt that anyone thinks tap water fits this definition. In addition to chlorine, which is used as a disinfectant, tap water also contains dioxins and carcinogens, such as trichloroethylene and triphenylmethane. Tap water meets certain levels of safety for these substances, but it still contains toxins.

Tap water is sterilized with chlorine, which can kill bacteria in the water. But when chlorine is added to water, large amounts of free radicals are produced. Microorganisms die as a result of those free radicals and, therefore, people consider that sterilized water "clean." But although microorganisms die when this kind of sterilization is used, the tap water involved gets oxidized.

The level of oxidation in water can be measured with something called the "oxidation-reduction electrical potential." Oxidation, which is bad for water, is the process in which electrons either break away or get taken away from molecules. Reduction, which is good, is the opposite, in which electrons are received by molecules. Based on the measurement of these fluctuating electrons, one can determine whether the water at hand will oxidize or reduce other substances. Therefore, the lower the electrical potential, the stronger the reduction power of the water will be (i.e., the power to reduce other substances); while water with higher electrical potential will be more likely to oxidize other substances. So, how does one find "good" water with a high reduction power?

You can use electrical means to create water with strong reduction capability ("kangen water"). Purification devices exist that ionize and create this type of water through electrolysis.

Alkaline ion purifiers and minus ion purifiers also use the same mechanism to produce water with reduction power, but when electrolysis occurs in these devices, minerals such as calcium and magnesium from the water attach themselves to the cathodes. Therefore, water that has been electrically treated can collect more minerals. Furthermore, when electrolysis occurs, active hydrogen is also produced, serving to remove excess free radicals from the body. When water passes through these purifiers, chlorine and chemical substances found in tap water get removed. The result is what I call "good water," pure, clean, alkaline water with plenty of minerals.

Recently, people have begun talking about small water molecules called "clusters" as being a requirement for good water. But at present, opinions are divided over the pros and cons of these clusters, so there is still no clear understanding of this matter.

To put it another way, good water means water with strong reduction power that has not been polluted with chemical substances.

There are many brands of mineral water, both domestic and imported. Among minerals found in water, calcium and magnesium are especially important for humans. In fact, the balance of these two minerals is very important. Calcium that enters the body does not go to fluids outside cells, but instead, remains within cells. When calcium collects inside cells, it becomes a cause of arteriosclerosis and high blood pressure. However, if the right amount of magnesium is consumed at the same time, it can prevent the excess accumulation of calcium in cells. The appropriate ratio of calcium to magnesium is said to be 2 to 1. Deep ocean water, which contains a lot of magnesium and hard water, can also be called "good water, because in addition to magnesium and calcium, it also contains iron, copper, fluorine and other minerals."

Incidentally, the hardness of water can be determined using the following formula:

(Calcium amount x 2.5) + (magnesium amount x 4.1) = hardness.

If the mineral value of water is below 100, it is considered "soft water," and anything over 100 is called "hard water." But one thing you must be careful of with these mineral waters is that if they are left in PET/plastic bottles for too long, their reduction power gradually decreases.

Moreover, if all your drinking water is bottled mineral water, it will cost time and money to buy enough. In order to drink plenty of good water everyday, even using it for cooking, I believe it is necessary to buy and use a purifier that has strong reduction power.

Also, when cold water is consumed, your body tries to heat the water as fast as it can, using various means so as to bring that temperature up to the same level as the temperature of your body. In fact, drinking water and stimulating the sympathetic nerves is one part of the system of producing energy to raise your body temperature.

However, keep in mind that trying to increase energy consumption by drinking water, like ice water, that is too cold, will have the opposite effect. This happens because water that is too cold cools the body at once, causing diarrhea and other physical problems.

Lately, there has been an increase in the number of people, especially young people, with "low body temperature syndrome" in which one's average body temperature is around 95°F. This low body temperature can have various harmful effects. A healthy person's normal body temperature is about 98.6°F, but once this falls, the rate of metabolism declines by as much as 50%. Furthermore, the body temperature at which cancer cells can multiply more easily is around 95°F. This is because the activity of enzymes becomes slower, decreasing the body's immune functions. Enzymes work more actively in higher body temperature. People get fevers because their bodies are actually trying to increase their immune functions. Thus, unless it is summertime, it is safer to drink water that is around 68°F.

DRINK A LOT OF GOOD WATER TO LOSE WEIGHT

When you walk around New York City, you frequently come across obese people walking around carrying bottled water. That is because drinking plenty of water is thought to be effective for their diet. The idea of losing weight just by drinking water may sound bogus, but the idea holds some truth.

When you drink water, the sympathetic nerves get stimulated, activating energy metabolism and increasing caloric consumption, which results in weight loss. When you stimulate the sympathetic nerves, adrenaline is secreted. Adrenaline activates the hormone-sensitive lipase found in fat tissue, which then breaks down triglycerides into fatty acid and glycerol, making it easier for your body to burn stored fat.

There have been reports showing how much caloric consumption increases as a result of drinking water. According to these reports, consistently drinking a little over two cups of water three times a day increases the number of calories burned in the body by approximately 30%. Moreover, about 30 minutes after drinking water, the calorie burn rate reaches its peak.

This fact makes it clear that people with excess fat should make it a habit to drink at least 6.5 cups of good water every day. And what kind of water is most effective for this purpose? Water that is lower in temperature than your body temperature but not icy cold. According to experiments, cold water that is about 70°F will increase caloric consumption. Cold water is considered good because considerable amounts of energy get used to warm up that water to body temperature.

The human body is equipped with various means for stabilizing body temperature. For example, when you go to the bathroom and urinate on a cold morning, you get a shiver. That is because warm urine, which had accumulated in the bladder, is suddenly lost from the body, resulting in shivering in order to quickly recover some of the heat.

PREVENT OVEREATING WITH ENZYMES

No matter how often you drink good water, you should not expect significant weight loss until your eating habits also change. Changing your eating habits does not necessarily mean decreasing the amount you eat. It is important to eat foods rich in enzymes if you want to lose your extra weight.

If you eat only foods containing a lot of enzymes, your body naturally adjusts its weight to what is most suited for you. People gain excess weight from eating foods that are oxidized and processed foods that have lost all their enzymes. They experience hunger pangs because they are not eating foods that contain nutrients the body really needs—the vitamins, minerals and enzymes. These people are not eating because they need more food; rather, they eat to satiate their body's craving for enzymes and trace nutrients like vitamins and minerals. You can only make hunger pangs disappear by eating good foods, foods abundant in enzymes.

There are people who, even if they have enough enzymes, feel hungry because they are lacking trace nutrients. Although trace nutrients are mainly vitamins and minerals, there are also indispensable substances called "coenzymes" which ensure that enzymes are working sufficiently in the body.

Recently coenzyme Q10 has been attracting attention as something good for your health and figure. However, Q10 is not the only necessary coenzyme for humans.

The number of coenzymes that are needed is actually fairly small. In the past, a well-balanced meal would have provided you with enough trace nutrients. But recently, the amount of trace nutrients found in fruits and vegetables has been on the decline, If your hunger pangs do not go away even if you switch over to a well-balanced diet, you should take supplements containing trace nutrients.

When trying to lose weight, you should consider not just the amount of food you need, but also how and when you eat it. Most overweight people do not chew well. For that reason, they eat their meals faster, raising their blood sugar level, and before their satiety center can send out a signal telling the person that they are full, they end up overeating. Just by chewing each mouthful 30-50 times, you will naturally start to eat less.

If food is still left in your stomach when you go to sleep, whether carbohydrates or proteins, most of it will be converted into fat by insulin.

In America, low-carb diets have gained popularity. With this diet, you eat few or no carbohydrates. But experimental results have shown that even if you have a low-carb, high-protein diet, if you continue to eat late at night, you will gain weight just as if you ate carbs. This is because a person who eats just before going to bed secretes large amounts of insulin, storing all the food as fat. In other words, unless you change your other eating habits, not only are low-carb diets ineffective, but your body will become acidic, increasing the possibility of getting osteoporosis and other diseases.

On the other hand, a person who is too thin does not secrete enough insulin, resulting in food getting excreted from the body undigested and unabsorbed. In other words, although the results are the exact opposite of each other, the cause of being overweight or underweight is the same.

If you eat enzyme-rich food the proper way and drink the necessary amount of good water, there is no need to go on a diet to lose or gain weight. Your body will adjust itself to its most suitable weight. As proof of this, if a person who is too thin follows this health lifestyle, he or she will actually gain weight to become normal size.

If you master habits that are good for your health and continue following the Enzyme Factor Diet and Lifestyle on a daily basis, your body will naturally assume the right condition.

THE GROUNDBREAKING METHOD TO IMPROVE BOWEL FUNCTION

Health-wise, one of the most troubling conditions for many women is constipation. And quite a few people take laxatives almost on a daily basis.

However, I believe much medication is something akin to poison. The more your intestine gets stimulated with drugs, the more it will require stronger stimulation. Those who take laxatives may know this, because in the beginning, you may have had to take only one pill to produce a bowel movement, but with repeated doses, the laxative becomes less effective, requiring you to increase the drug to two pills, then three, or switching to a different laxative in the hope that it will work better.

Constipation is one of the causes of bad intestinal characteristics; thus it is necessary to alleviate this condition as soon as possible. No matter how good the food is, if you cannot excrete that food properly, it will rot and produce toxins in the intestine. Once it reaches this state, the balance of the intestinal bacterial flora will collapse in an instant. The reason you get pimples and rashes when you are constipated is that toxins, which get produced in the intestine, cannot be sufficiently excreted from the intestine.

Needless to say, the most desirable situation is to have well-regulated bowel movements in a natural condition. In order to do that, in addition to eating foods rich in enzymes, it is important to stimulate the intestine by eating foods abundant in dietary fibers, drinking plenty of good water, massaging your stomach along the flow of your intestine and strengthening your abdominal muscles.

If, after doing all this you do not see much improvement, I would recommend having an enema. What I recommend is a coffee enema, which involves cleaning the colon with water containing coffee plus minerals and lactobacilli-creating extracts.

Many people in Japan worry that if they have enemas, it will become a habit, and the colon will eventually be unable to work on its own. But according to my clinical data, there is no need to worry. Rather, people who regularly administer their own enemas have better functioning intestines and cleaner intestinal characteristics, free of stagnant stool and impacted feces.

In contrast, for people who habitually use laxatives—whether chemical products, herbal medicine or natural herbal teas—their intestinal walls become discolored and black. And the more medication they take, the worse the state of their intestines becomes, gradually slowing down intestinal movement. When intestinal movement stops, it becomes easier for stagnant stool to remain in the intestine, creating problems.

I have a doctor friend who, despite his healthy body, still has coffee enemas twice a day. It is not because he cannot have bowel movements, but rather, because he inevitably has some food substances that have abnormally fermented or remain undigested in the colon, even with proper excretion. It is better for the body to excrete stool as soon as possible, especially from the left side of the colon where stool easily stagnates. Following my advice, it has been close to 20 years since my friend made a habit of using coffee enemas, but his physical condition is better now than it was before.

Even I often do coffee enemas. When I say cleansing the intestine, only the left side of the large intestine gets cleansed by the enema, so it will not hinder the functions of the small intestine, where digestion and absorption occur. Thus, you may have enemas free of worries.

What Lifestyle Habit Prevents the Exhaustion of Source enzymes?

Enzymes control all human life and life energy. Even the acts of waking up and falling asleep involve enzymes. If you go to sleep thinking what time you want to wake up the next day, you will often wake up the next morning around that time. That can be attributed to enzymes since the act of thinking itself is nothing more than enzymes working in the brain. Everything a person does, whether it is moving the hand or the eyes, or using the brain, depends on enzyme functions.

The human body is equipped to maintain homeostasis. A cut healing and skin returning to its normal color after getting tanned are examples of the body returning to homeostasis. The body's homeostatic functions respond sensitively to any abnormality and try to return the body to its original health and normal condition. That is why if you suddenly do strenuous exercises, or go to bed at 3:00 a.m. instead of the usual earlier time, or wake up at 4:00 a.m. instead of the usual 6:00 a.m., the body tries to adjust to these abnormalities. What helps the body regulate homeostasis is none other than enzymes.

If abnormalities occur once in awhile, the body will be able to adjust to them. However, if the abnormalities are repeated or continue, source enzymes get exhausted, collapsing the internal balance of the body's enzymes. This is why leading a well-regulated life means preventing the excess consumption of source enzymes.

People who stay up late or do other things that equate to leading an unhealthy life waste that many more source enzymes. I believe the actual cause of death from overworking is the total exhaustion of source enzymes.

Being a physician is a challenging job, but since taking up this profession 45 years ago, I have never missed work on account of my health. That is because I have mastered a lifestyle that does not exhaust my source enzymes. In discussing my lifestyle below, my intention is not for you to completely imitate me. Each person has his or her own individual life rhythm and mine may not be best for you.

But no matter what kind of rhythm you have, continuously leading a well-regulated life is absolutely necessary for maintaining your health. For that reason, I would be more than pleased if you are able to find some useful hints in my daily life activities.

MORNING

Waking up at 6 a.m., I start the day with light hand and feet exercises, which I do in bed. After lightly shaking my hands and feet, I get up from the bed, open the windows, and deeply inhale the fresh morning air. This enables me to replace with fresh air the stale air that had collected inside my lungs. Then I return to my bed. While lying on my back, I do some light exercises, alternately raising my arms, right and left, then alternately raising my legs and then lifting both arms and both legs. After that, I do something similar to calisthenic stretching, slowly activating my blood circulation and flow in the lymph nodes.

After I get my blood circulating, I get up from bed, and this time I do 100 karate thrusts each on the left and right, then five minutes of basic stretching.

After finishing my morning exercises, I go to the kitchen and slowly drink two or three cups of good water at about 70°F. About 20 minutes after drinking the water, just as the water is moving into the intestines, I eat fresh fruits rich with enzymes, followed by breakfast 30–40 minutes later.

The main thing I eat for breakfast is brown rice mixed with five, six, or seven types of grains. For side dishes, I have steamed vegetables, *natto* (fermented soybeans), *non* (dried seaweed) and a handful of reconstituted wakame seaweed.

AFTERNOON

A little after 11 a.m., I drink about two cups of water. Thirty minutes later, I eat fruits if available.

Incidentally many people eat fruit as a dessert, but I recommend eating fruit 30 minutes before meals as often as possible. Fresh fruit abundant in enzymes digests well and by eating it before meals, it helps the functions of the gastrointestinal system and raises the blood sugar level, thus preventing you from overeating.

Even during meals, if you eat things that have not been cooked, like salad, your digestion will be better. This is the reason salad is served first in a course meal, and animal proteins such as meat and fish are served as the main course. Since people cannot eat too many raw vegetables all at once, I frequently eat cooked vegetables as well. However, if you boil vegetables in water that is too hot, the enzymes will get lost. So I eat vegetables that have either been steamed or blanched for two minutes.

My lunch is mainly a packed lunch from home that I myself prepare. I do on occasion go out and enjoy lunch with my friends, but I basically eat my homemade lunch, consisting of brown rice with a variety of grains.

Following my meal, I take a nap for about 20–30 minutes. By resting a little bit, my morning fatigue disappears, and I can start my afternoon work with a clear head.

EVENING

After lunch, I try not to eat any snacks. When 4:30 p.m. comes around, I again drink two cups of water. I then wait another 30 minutes before eating fruit. 30-40 minutes after that, I have dinner.

I eat a lot of fruits everyday. I believe that a person should eat as much fruit as he or she wants.

For dinner, I eat my food made from fresh ingredients immediately after it is cooked, and I chew my food really well. What I have for dinner is not that different from my breakfast.

In my household, there is little conversation during meals. That is because we try to chew our food well. When we do talk, it is after we have completely swallowed our food. It is important to remember not to have anything in your mouth while talking. It is not only about manners: this prevents food from going down the wrong pipe and you from swallowing air with your food.

If you like to have a drink after dinner it is okay, but I try not to drink coffee or green tea if at all possible. Rather, I drink organic herbal tea, soba (buckwheat) tea or barley tea. However, regarding soba tea or barley tea, you have to remember that since these teas are roasted, they need to be properly preserved in a sealed container in order to prevent them from becoming oxidized. The truth is, it is better to drink tea right after it has been roasted, but since that is difficult to do in our busy daily life, you should keep only small amounts of tea and, if opened, finish drinking it as soon as possible.

After finishing my dinner around 6:00–6:30 p.m., I do not put any food or water in my mouth before going to bed five hours later. When I get thirsty during the summer months, I drink just enough good water to quench my thirst (approximately 1 cup) about one hour before I go to bed. But it is better to avoid drinking any water late at night.

Take Five-Minute Power Naps Regularly

After lunch, I make it my habit to nap for about 20–30 minutes, but when I feel tired at other times, I take five-minute power naps.

What is most important when taking a nap is resting in a relaxed position. I tend to rest on my stomach frequently, but if you are relaxed, you can also nap sitting in a chair with your legs raised.

You may wonder how you can get rid of your fatigue in only 20-30 minutes. It works because the short rest allows your body to balance itself — homeostasis. Rest and sleep return the weakened functions of your entire body, such as blood flow, lymph flow, the nervous system and internal secretions back to normal.

Why does rest improve your body's homeostasis? This is only my theory, but I believe the reason is as follows:

When you are awake and active, it means you are using many more enzymes. Thus if you are resting in a relaxed position, the various body functions are also resting during that time, and enzymes are not being used for activities or movement. The enzymes are free to work instead in those fatigued areas to help re-energize and restore homeostasis.

The fact is, if you rest for even five or ten minutes when you feel sleepy or tired, you will recover more quickly. If you continue to work when you are tired or drowsy, it will not improve your overall efficiency. Recently, workplaces have begun to recognize the effectiveness of napping, and some businesses have gone so far as to provide a place to power nap.

At my medical clinic, I have made the one hour between 12 p.m. and 1 p.m. a time for rest. As one would expect, since it is a clinic, not everyone is able to rest at the same time, so my staff eats lunch and takes naps in shifts. During that time, even if there is a phone call for the person who is resting, that person does not answer the phone unless it is an emergency. Thus, if you take a peek into the back of my clinic, you will see doctors and nurses taking power naps in any position they like.

Sleep plays an extremely important role in maintaining the human body's rhythm. It is understandable that a well-regulated life is synonymous with going to bed early and waking up early. If the following things are fixed, like what time you go to sleep and wake up, in addition to what time you take your meals and naps, the body's homeostasis will not be burdened, effectively preventing the excess consumption of source enzymes.

Currently, my biggest problem is jet lag. I basically live in New York, but I also go to Japan twice a year for two months at a time to work. However, I am always troubled by the time difference (13-14 hours) between New York and Japan.

Since my body's rhythm changes completely between day and night, it always takes my body about two weeks to get used to the new rhythm. I have observed that it takes about that much time for my body's kidney, liver and gastrointestinal functions to become completely readjusted.

When you feel naturally sleepy as a result of your body's rhythm, it is probably the best time for you to sleep. There are people who habitually take sleeping pills because they cannot sleep, but these drugs have a direct effect on the brain, so they are very dangerous. Sleeping pills exhaust large numbers of enzymes in the brain, which could predispose the person to senility or Alzheimer's. If you regularly use sleeping pills and notice that you have been getting more forgetful recently, this is a dangerous signal. Medication, under any circumstances, must not be taken casually.

You do not need medicine if you live a well-regulated life and take power naps when you get sleepy during the day. Your body's homeostasis will be in balance, and you will eventually be able to sleep naturally at night.

TOO MUCH EXERCISE HAS NO BENEFITS
AND CAUSES MUCH HARM

Moderate exercise is necessary in order to lead a healthy life. As described earlier, I also do my own version of exercises every morning.

There are five "flows" in the human body: blood and lymph flow, gastrointestinal flow, urine flow, air flow and internal energy flow ("chi"). It is important that these "flows" are not interrupted, and the thing that allows these flows to continue unhindered is exercise.

By moving your entire body, your blood circulation and lymph flow improve. This activates your body's metabolism, which in turn, allows indispensable vitamins and minerals to be supplied to your entire body more easily, thus creating an environment more conducive to the work of enzymes. As a result, the functions of your whole body improve.

However, this is only the case when you exercise in the right amount.

Too much exercise can actually damage your health, because the more you exercise, the more free radicals you produce in your body. This, I believe, is why we often see cases where a person dies suddenly from heart failure while jogging. Many women jog every day, but young female runners in their twenties who run close to 10km (6 miles) a day become extremely skinny and have flat chests and buttocks. In some cases their menstrual cycle stops. This is because their bodies are not producing enough female hormones.

Your body's homeostasis collapses when you overdo things. Moderation is one important key to health. Moderation, in this case, does not mean half-heartedly doing something, but rather, it means doing exercise most suitable for your physical condition, lifestyle, and mental health. This is why moderation differs from person to person. The moderate exercise I do every morning was created by putting together many things I had tested myself. If people who have never moved their bodies begin to exercise the way I do, they will stress their muscles or joints. Since stress produces large amounts of free radicals in the body, exercise that causes stress will have no health benefits.

As I have already stated, moderation is different for every person. Based on that assumption, I would say that, generally speaking, it is ideal to walk about a mile or two every day at your own pace. One benefit of exercising is that it improves the airflow in your lungs. When there is better airflow, fresh air enters your body, activating your metabolism and improving your body's blood, lymph, and gastrointestinal flow.

Another good thing to do when you have spare time is to close your eyes and take several deep breaths. By taking deep breaths, you can take in the necessary oxygen without exercising excessively. Moreover, inhaling deeply also has the effect of stimulating parasympathetic nerves, stabilizing your mental state, and heightening your body's immune functions.

By all means, exercise every day, but exercise in moderation so that you can continue to enjoy exercising every day without too much stress.

HOW CHAPLIN WAS ABLE TO HAVE CHILDREN AT AGE 73

There is also one other thing that is essential when talking about healthy lifestyles, and that is one's sex life.

Recently, even young married couples have been reporting problems related to sex, such as lack of sex, erectile dysfunction, and infertility.

I believe that health, in the real sense, is when the various functions of your body, including your sex life, are regularly active.

Even many healthy people, when they enter their sixties and are asked about their sex lives, respond, "I don't have that kind of ability anymore," or "I no longer have any interest in that." But that is very unnatural from the medical point of view. I believe that a normal, healthy person's sex life ends at death.

However, if talking about the body's functions in this regard, a man who is really healthy can have morning erections everyday until the age of 75. A healthy woman may have regular periods until the age of 55.

The reason women reach this stage at a comparatively young age of 55 has largely to do with giving birth. Being pregnant means creating another person inside the body, thus greatly stressing the mother's body. A person needs youthfulness to endure that kind of physical stress. Childbirth is in itself a life-threatening event, but that risk increases the older one gets. The mother's calcium steadily gets depleted, and her body consumes enzymes for two instead of just herself. The body's ability to restore its source enzymes also decreases with age.

A person's body functions decline with age no matter what. Perhaps the body changes its hormonal balance midway through life so that we can start to enjoy living our lives for ourselves. Let's say a woman lives to be 100. Her body's hormonal balance changes at the halfway point when she is 50, thus telling her that the time period for reproducing is over. I believe this is actually one of the body's defense mechanisms.

In the case of men, because they do not face big physical risks like pregnancy or childbirth, they can maintain the ability to reproduce for a longer period of time than women. If the men are healthy, their production of sperm can continue for a lifetime.

The painter Pablo Picasso, known to have energetically contributed to the artistic world even at 90, fathered a child at age 67. The famous comedic movie actor Charlie Chaplin married four times, and his last child was born when he was 73. The Japanese actor Uehara Ken fathered a child a decade ago at age 71, and the kabuki actor Nakamura Tomijyuro became a father at 74.

But please do not misunderstand me. I am not promoting the idea of older people having children. I am merely trying to make the point that your body's ability to reproduce is connected to the maintenance of your health. What the aforementioned four people had in common were healthy bodies and long, active careers.

Of course, enzymes have a big effect on one's sex life. A lifestyle that does not needlessly exhaust source enzymes is unmistakably connected to maintaining one's sexual functions.

POST-MENOPAUSE IS THE START OF GREAT SEX

The good news for post-menopausal women is that fertility and desire for sex are two entirely different issues.

It is true that once menstruation stops, women secrete fewer female hormones, resulting in physical changes such as insufficient vaginal lubrication and hair loss. But instead of seeing these changes in a negative light, think of this period as finally being free from menstruation and worry about getting pregnant. The post-menopausal years are a time when you can have the best sex of your life. Your new freedom allows you to fully enjoy sex mentally and physically.

Once men and women both reach an age where hormonal balances change, their sexual desire declines. However, it is important for both women and men to continue enjoying their sex lives even if with less frequency.

With a little effort, men can improve their sexual functions without depending on drugs. The easiest way is to drink two cups of water about one hour before sex. Once you have drunk the water, the fluid collects in the bladder, stimulating the prostate and increasing erection remarkably. Incidentally, this effect is not attained by drinking beer or tea, because caffeine and alcohol constrict blood vessels.

Many older men will say, "I do not feel like doing something so troublesome and tiring," but for a married couple or a man and woman who truly love each other, sex should never be a tiring or exhausting act. It is also medically proven that being mentally and physically happy enhances a person's immune functions. Every man would like to always be his young and vibrant self, desirable and loved by a woman. And every woman would also like to be beautiful, desirable and loved by a man. It is very important to continue having those feelings in order to live a long and healthy life.

This is true of everything; the person who gives up first loses. If you give up on things mentally, your body will age that much faster. Never give up. That is the secret to living a long and healthy life.

Chapter 4

Pay Attention to Your "Script of Life"

In the past 100 years, medicine has made rapid progress. Ironically, the number of people who get sick has continued to rise every year. If medicine has really progressed, why aren't there fewer sick people?

Is it because modern medicine is mistaken in its basic premise? I believe the answer is yes. Prevalent medical theory states that bacteria and viruses are the cause of contagious diseases. But this is a one-sided view. We must be mindful that we develop diseases by allowing our bodies to be hosts to those bacteria and viruses. Modern medicine is based on the idea of treating, or curing, diseases, while true medicine should be based on the idea of *maintaining one's health.*

I began seriously researching the relationship between food and health almost 40 years ago. At that time, having examined many stomachs and intestines of Americans and finding that gastrointestinal characteristics are very good barometers of health, I realized that improving them is the shortcut to promoting good health. Thus, while I tried to develop and propagate the technique of colonoscopic polypectomy in order to help people suffering from illnesses, I continued to search for their root causes.

I read many articles and scientific reports, collected clinical data with the cooperation of my patients, used my own body to verify the influence of drugs, and even studied animals in the wild. The result I arrived at was that if you go against the laws of nature, which encompass everything in this world (one could also say God's will), you will become sick. Humans are a part of nature, not separate from it, and without it we cannot achieve health and continued existence. Like other animals, humans must consume foods suitable to the specifications of their own species and the environment in which they live. The basic principle of human life is to eat plants and animals that occur naturally in their region. For humans used to a diet consisting of grains, vegetables, sea vegetables, fruits and fish, excess quantities of chemical-laden meat, milk and highly-processed, enzyme-poor foods cannot be digested.

I believe we are all capable of living full, healthy lives. It is true that some people, having had the misfortune to be born with congenital diseases, are destined to struggle with health issues much of their lives. Some of these people have experienced negative hereditary or environmental influences in utero, while the causes of other congenital diseases are not yet understood. Yet I believe even people with chronic hereditary diseases can improve their overall health with good living habits.

Everyone Is Meant to Live a Full Life

Are we all not born with "life scripts" for living healthy lives? Animals instinctively know what they need to do in order to survive. Wild animals understand their own life scripts and try to follow those scripts. The teeth of carnivores and herbivores are different because that is how nature tells them what type of food they should eat.

The alignment and ratio of our teeth, is also a perfect example of nature's law at work. It means that we, humans, also have our own scripts for vital good health, but in our arrogance we often ignore them. One reason for this is human greed. Our ability to think, given to us by the grace of God, has been misinterpreted by many to mean that humans are special beings of a higher class than animals. We breed and control animals in a manner convenient to us. Our desire to eat delicious things has led us to eat "foods" not found in nature. Our desire to live more comfortable lives with modern conveniences has led us to destroy much of the natural environment. Our desire to grow crops with greater ease has led to the use of agricultural chemicals. Our desire for more land and money has led to discord and disputes. Perhaps, humans today are paying for their continuously expanding greed in the form of disease.

But it is also about time that modern medicine realized its errors. We humans are also a part of nature. In order for us to live healthily, we must follow nature's laws. Entrusting oneself to nature's law means listening to one's inherent life script. An overweight person feels hungry because he or she lacks necessary nutrients. A person with diarrhea or constipation is not eating foods suitable to that person's digestive system. And we fall ill when we ignore nature's laws.

Thus, I am convinced that medicine in the future should focus on the laws of nature. We must pay attention to the script nature has written for humans, try to awaken our inherent ability to cure ourselves, and shift to the promotion of health instead of trying to forcefully suppress illnesses.

SPECIALIZATION IS RUINING MEDICINE

The first step towards following the laws of nature is to stop the practice of healthcare specialization. Medical specialization makes us unable to see the forest for the trees. Nothing in nature stands by itself. Everything influences and maintains balance with everything else.

There has been a recent movement in Japan to "plant a forest to grow an ocean." This is a project started by fishermen who, wondering why fish were suddenly disappearing from the ocean, discovered that several years earlier a large number of mountain trees had been cut down for development. They found a connection between these logging activities and the decline in fish population. The fishermen's project aims to replant trees in the mountains in order to "bring back" the fish. At first glance, it may seem like there is little relation between trees on the mountain and fish in the ocean, but in the circle of nature, the two things are closely interconnected.

Similarly, the separate activities of 60 trillion cells, carrying out the five flows in the human body — blood and lymph, gastrointestinal, urine, air, and energy — are all closely intertwined. A problem in one will impact the health of all. Ignoring this interconnection and trying to treat only individual organs constitutes a failure to see the big picture. If specialization of medical treatment progresses at the rate it is presently moving, in the near future we will no longer have real physicians. We will be left with only specialists who understand their specific area of specialization but cannot address the condition of their patients' health as a whole.

Even if just by looking at the eyes and complexion of a patient it is clear that he or she has some physical ailment, a gastrointestinal specialist might simply perform a colonoscopy and, upon finding no polyps, tell the patient, "Congratulations, you're fine. There were no polyps or cancer." This is quite irresponsible, as a simple colonoscopic examination by itself cannot assess the overall health of that person.

There are some who call me "the number one gastrointestinal surgical endoscopist in America," but I do not think I have an exceptional talent. I am only trying to treat my patients every day by paying careful attention to their bodies.

Currently in America, it has become common practice for breast cancer patients to receive colon examinations. I was actually the one to first publish this idea. At the time, I was praised for this discovery, but, frankly speaking, I believe another doctor would have realized the same thing if he or she had been trained to regard a patient's body as a whole unified organism.

When I meet a person who has cancer, I know they have cancer without having to look inside their bodies. It is hard to explain in words, but I get a feeling as if my "chi" (energy) is being sucked out of me. When I speak about things like this, most doctors smile wryly. However, this is not simply my imagination, but a physical sensation backed by my long-term clinical experience.

I once had a 38-year-old female patient who complained, "Doctor, I have cancer here," while pointing to her upper abdominal area. I also had the same feeling. However, prior to her coming to see me, she had already been to many doctors and had undergone many tests, but everywhere she went, the test results came back "normal." Even after I carefully examined her endoscopically, I still could not see any signs of cancer anywhere. I did not think there was much to worry about since she was young, but because she persistently complained about there being something wrong, I put a contrast dye from the duodenum into the bile duct and did an x-ray examination. (The bile duct cannot be examined endoscopically because it is extremely thin.) Tests such as putting contrast dye into the bile duct are not commonly done.

Using this test, I found cancer the size of the tip of a pinky in the bile duct.

Another patient came to me for a consultation saying he was sure he had stomach cancer. This person always had normal endoscopic examination results. But in this case as well, because the patient persistently complained and since I also had the strange sensation there was something wrong, I decided to reexamine him two months after the consultation. When I reexamined him, I found a small ulcer in the stomach. Upon taking a biopsy and testing the tissue sample, we discovered that a scirrhous carcinoma had developed and had already spread under the stomach mucosa. In addition to being a type of cancer that progresses very quickly, scirrhous carcinoma is extremely difficult to detect. It is very hard to find endoscopically once it has developed under the mucosa, making this a terrifying disease. If I had not reexamined him when I did, the cancer would have killed him.

The time a doctor spends with a patient face-to-face is not very long. During that short period of time, the doctor concentrates on looking for an SOS signal that the patient's body is emitting. Unfortunately however, there are only a few doctors who are willing to pay attention to the patient's whole body, because healthcare has become completely specialized.

I am sure you have experienced this before, but prior to receiving any medical examination, you (the patient) must first decide which doctor you would like to consult. In the exam room, the doctor will ask you,

"So what brings you here today?" And if the patient says, "My stomach hurts," they then get their stomach examined. If nothing abnormal is found in the stomach, they are sent home with an "Ok, there's nothing wrong with you" stamp of approval. Unless the patient asks for more testing to be done, the consultation will end at that point. In the case of bad doctors, they may simply ignore the patient's request and say, "It's all in your imagination. There is no need for that kind of test" and send the patient away.

But, as I have previously stated, I believe it is necessary for doctors to listen to their patients and take seriously what their patients tell them. I am very saddened by the present situation of the specialized healthcare system because I strongly believe that individuals cannot truly become doctors in this way. What is more unfortunate is that MDs are no longer required to do a year of internship before they specialize. This means they are not given an adequate chance to learn about parts of the body other than those in their area of specialty.

At my New York clinic, in order to alleviate my patients' anxiety, I perform a general examination of the entire body. First, before performing an esophagogastroduodenoscopy (EGD) or a colonoscopy, I examine my patient's skin condition, blood pressure, pulse, oxygen saturation level, thyroid glands, lymph glands, abnormalities in the joints and muscles, and a breast examination in women.

If my patient is a female, I ask her if she would like me to check her cervix for possible cervical cancer. If she agrees, I examine the cervix using the colonoscope. The cervical examination usually takes less than a minute, and my patients end up very happy because they do not have to make a separate trip to the gynecologist.

Although I am a gastrointestinal specialist, I also examine the prostate and breasts just as I examine the cervix. My patients are happy with these examinations, and it becomes a very good learning experience for me as a physician.

CHOOSE TO BE HEALTHY 10 YEARS FROM NOW, RATHER THAN HAVING A STEAK TONIGHT

I can learn many things from examining a single illness.

For example, during breast cancer examinations, I ask my patients about their dietary history. From such interviews, I can find causal relationships between diet and illness. I have discovered that women with breast cancer love to drink coffee, frequently consume dairy products like milk, cheese and yogurt and have a diet mainly consisting of meats. For many people who have this kind of diet, even if they have not yet developed breast cancer, their breasts feel very cystic, a condition called fibrocystic disease. The cause of fibrocystic disease is the combination of dairy products and a meat diet, and if the patient's dietary habits do not improve, her chances of developing breast cancer are quite high.

Thus, I strongly advise people with fibrocystic disease to improve their dietary habits immediately. When I ask women with fibrocystic disease, "You like coffee, dairy products and meat, don't you?" they are usually very surprised that I know this. After I discuss my clinical data, dietary suggestions and reasoning for my suggestions, most people decide to change their dietary habits.

My medical treatment is based on things I have learned from examining many patients. Likewise, my suggestions for a proper lifestyle are also based on my observations of various patients. Along with changing one's diet, massaging the breast about five minutes everyday has shown to be helpful in preventing breast cancer, something I have learned from clinical observation.

I do not know if breast cancer specialists suggest these preventative measures to their patients. But when I see my patients one year after I give them this advice, their breast tissues are in fact much softer, and their fibrocystic condition is often cured.

What makes me most happy as a doctor is not curing diseases or being called a skilled physician, but being able to give accurate advice to people with "dormant illnesses" and helping them become healthy.

After so many years in this field, it is no wonder that I have become keenly aware of the importance of daily diet. However, today there are many kinds of food widely considered "good" that are actually harmful to the body. During the past 30 years, I have constantly lectured and attended public forums as well as talking with patients both in the USA and in Japan about the relationship between diet and health and the kinds of food that are dangerous. But changing socially accepted norms has not been easy. Furthermore, if the specialization of healthcare progresses at this rate, it will become increasingly difficult for young doctors to learn the things that I and many other older physicians have learned from clinical experience.

What we need in the future is preventive medicine. And in order to institute correct preventive medicine, proper knowledge about diet is indispensable. Yet it is very hard to reform the mind of an adult whose existing "common sense" is already set. It might be different if that person were sick, but if the person has only a latent illness, the choice would be to have a steak tonight over being healthy 10 years from now. For those of you who have read this book up to this point, I am hoping that you will choose the "being healthy" option.

My focus now is on educating the next generation. We often hear about educating the whole person intellectually, physically, and spiritually. But what I am hoping to incorporate is diet education, helping people gain correct knowledge about food. The lunches currently served in schools are often based on mistaken ideas and calorie calculations that are very dangerous. Thus, I believe school lunch reform and diet education targeting children should be the most urgent task at present.

HUMANS ARE ABLE TO LIVE BECAUSE OF MICROORGANISMS

Have you ever thought about what happens to fish that die in the ocean? When you look at the bottom of the ocean, you will not find any accumulation of fish carcasses. So where do the fish remains go? They actually disappear. Microorganisms in the ocean slowly break them down, and they disappear without much notice.

Although we cannot see them with our naked eye, our world is full of microorganisms. Even in clean air, it is said there are about 100 microorganisms within a radius of 1 cm from any given point. Even at over six miles in the air and six miles underground, there are microorganisms. Of course there are many microorganisms in the sea as well. Even inside human intestines, there are many microorganisms called intestinal bacterial flora. In other words, we are living in a soup of microorganisms.

There are about 300 different types and a total of about 1,000 trillion intestinal bacteria living inside each human intestine. But they are not there without a purpose. Many things that go on inside our bodies are done by these bacteria. The most important function these bacteria fulfill is to create source enzymes that become the source of our life energy. Intestinal bacteria are believed to create approximately 3,000 types of enzymes.

Among intestinal bacteria, there are bad bacteria and good bacteria. In general, we call bacteria like the lactobacilli, which work productively for humans, "good bacteria," and those that cause decay and otherwise harmfully affect the human body "bad bacteria."

Good bacteria, in a word, are bacteria with antioxidant enzymes. When free radicals are produced in the intestine, these bacteria die and produce antioxidant enzymes, thus neutralizing the free radicals.

There are countless small projections called villi in the intestine. Lactobacilli, which are good bacteria, enter the spaces between those villi projections. Many cells involved in the immune system, like white blood cells and natural killer cells, are produced in these villi. When these white blood cells and natural killer cells fight foreign bodies such as proteins, bacteria, viruses and cancer cells, large numbers of free radicals are produced. The lactobacilli play an active role in the removal of these free radicals.

It is my belief that the free radicals that could not be neutralized because of the lack of "good bacteria" or some other reason cause inflammation of the extremely delicate villi, destroying the villi and causing ulcerative colitis or Crohn's disease.

On the other hand, bad bacteria work to decay indigestible matter and are generally thought to be toxic. But by causing the abnormal fermentation of indigestible matter and creating toxic gases, they stimulate the intestine to excrete gas and stool, thus helping to remove the indigestible matter from the body as quickly as possible. Thus, I believe you cannot clearly distinguish or designate intestinal bacteria as good or bad. "Bad bacteria" may also exist in the body for a particular purpose that is not necessarily harmful.

In addition to good and bad bacteria, there are also bacteria that are neither toxic nor helpful. These are called "intermediate" or neutral bacteria. This, again, is not a very precise way to classify these bacteria. What is important is the balance of all of these different types of bacteria. As with protein, no matter how important the nutrient, if you consume too much of it, it will become poisonous to your body. The same can be said of bad bacteria. If the bad bacteria increase too much, they could cause problems, even if they are of a type of bacteria that your body needs in order to maintain its health.

It is all a matter of balance, and, as I have previously mentioned, the balance of intestinal bacteria is very delicate. Microorganisms are extremely fragile and are easily influenced by their environment. If the environment is suitable for propagation, they will increase several thousand, even several million times over. But, if the environment is bad, they will die out very quickly.

The characteristic of intermediate bacteria is still unclear because, if surrounded by mostly good bacteria, they too will start producing antioxidant enzymes. But if surrounded by mostly bad bacteria, they too will start producing oxidized enzymes, transforming themselves into bacteria that are bad. In other words, intermediate bacteria are strongly influenced by whatever bacteria are surrounding them.

People dislike bad bacteria, but we ourselves create the intestinal environments conducive to them. We cannot blame the microorganisms for our ignorance regarding dietary and lifestyle habits. Whether we transform the intermediate bacteria in our bodies into good or bad ones depends on our own actions.

CREATING AN INTESTINAL ENVIRONMENT CONDUCIVE FOR GOOD BACTERIA

Although enzymes are indispensable, the number of enzymes people can produce may be predetermined. I believe a person's life ends when the enzymes in the body are used up. Thinking of it in this way, it would not be a mistake to say source enzymes determine the span of our lives.

More than anything else, free radicals exhaust these precious enzymes. Modern society itself presents an environment where free radicals are easily produced. Stress, air pollution, ultraviolet rays, electromagnetic waves, bacterial or viral infections, exposure to x-ray or radiation are all factors that create free radicals.

However, in addition to these external factors, other activities produce free radicals, but we can easily avoid them if we're willing to make some lifestyle changes. Drinking, smoking, and the consumption of food additives, and oxidized food are all such preventable causes of damaging free radicals. Since these habits exhaust a huge number of enzymes, you are likely to become sick in time, unless you make a conscious effort to eliminate these activities.

If the number of enzymes in our bodies are already predetermined, we must depend on intestinal bacteria to produce additional enzymes to supplement our own. Thus, the only way we can increase our body's enzymes is by creating an intestinal environment conducive to good bacteria with their antioxidant enzymes.

When I tell people to eat foods rich in enzymes, it is because these foods allow good bacteria to propagate, thus becoming the raw material for enzymes.

Just as you see in nature, the accumulation of good things will eventually lead to a positive cycle. If you eat good food, drink good water, and continue to pursue a good lifestyle, your intestinal environment will naturally be well regulated, giving rise to an abundance of enzymes and allowing you to live a life filled with vitality.

On the other hand, disrupting this good cycle with a single bad habit can easily turn it into a bad cycle. If you continue to consume an animal diet of meat and dairy products, it will adversely impact your ability to digest and absorb nutrients, damaging your intestinal environment over time. If your intestinal environment deteriorates, your good bacteria will disappear and the intermediate bacteria will start changing into bad bacteria. This will create an environment in which your body can no longer neutralize free radicals. Furthermore, because your digestive ability deteriorates, the undigested food will start to rot in your intestines. Using that decaying food as nutrition, bad bacteria will begin producing a lot of toxic gases.

People who frequently pass unusually smelly gas have this bad cycle in their intestines. Infants who drink breast milk do not have odorous stool because they are consuming only living food. The stool of children raised on cow's milk has a more pungent smell.

Although your immune system also battles the toxins inside your intestine, there are hardly any good bacteria left to neutralize the free radicals that are produced from this battle. The result is, you cannot stop the bad effects of free radicals, and intestinal walls that have been destroyed by free radicals give rise to polyps and cancer.

You can reverse this cycle and create a good intestinal environment by paying closer attention to your diet and lifestyle. You have to make quite an effort to start the good cycle and keep it going, but once the good cycle starts, even if you eat a little meat and drink some alcohol once a month, your source enzymes that have been saved until then will compensate for the occasional lapses.

THE INSEPARABLE RELATIONSHIP BETWEEN OUR BODIES AND THE LAND

Americans have been eating an animal diet much longer than the Japanese, and the intestinal balance of Americans does not become as disrupted by eating meat as easily as the intestinal balance in Japanese people. I have often wondered why there is such a difference between these two groups. There are a couple of reasons I can think of.

First, the dietary culture cultivated over many years in each country differs.

Westerners have consumed a meat diet over the course of centuries, but the Japanese only adopted a meat diet during the Meiji Period (1868–1912), a relatively recent phenomenon. The intestines of Japanese who have been eating a diet mainly consisting of grains and vegetables for centuries, is 1.2 times as long as the intestines of Westerners in proportion to body size. Because their intestines are longer, it takes longer for their food to be excreted. Since the food stays in the body longer, the effect a meat diet has on their intestines is that much greater.

The other difference is found in the soil. The human body and land have an inseparable connection. We are now able to eat foods from around the world, but we still mostly eat food from the land where we live. Therefore, the health of people will depend largely on the condition of the land where they live.

This is a story from years ago, but the first time I saw vegetables sold in America, I was surprised by their size. Japanese vegetables, whether an eggplant or cucumber, are clearly smaller. I thought this was because the vegetables were all of a different type. But in fact, if you plant Japanese vegetable seeds in America, the vegetables will grow to be much bigger than if they had been grown in Japan. This is because American soil contains more calcium, minerals and vitamins than Japanese soil. For example, there is 3-5 times more calcium in spinach grown in America than in the spinach grown in Japan.

Another example is broccoli. According to some data I have seen, there are 178 milligrams of calcium in 100 grams of American broccoli. In contrast, there are only 57 milligrams of calcium in the same 100 grams of broccoli in Japan.

My theory is that although Americans have a diet centered on meat, their bodies are not as badly affected by this as Japanese people's because they eat vegetables grown on land rich in nutrients, thus allowing them to neutralize, to a certain degree, the slightly acidic pH balance of their bodies caused by the meat.

Years ago, there was a clear difference in the physical build between Japanese and Americans. However, Japanese bodies today are much bigger than before, and the cause is thought to be the general shift toward a Western diet. In other words, Japanese dietary habits and physique have changed with the import of a dietary culture consisting of meat, milk, cheese and butter.

Even so, if the Japanese want to become westernized in these ways, there is just one thing that cannot be changed, and that is Japanese soil. The richness of soil cannot be imitated as much as they try. One can say that the richness of soil is determined by the number of small animals and microorganisms that inhabit that soil. But in Japan, the land mostly originates from volcanic remains and does not contain as many nutrients for soil bacteria.

Thus, Japan's soil is not very rich in nutrients to begin with. Japanese people were able to maintain balance in their diet and health in the past because they ate grains and vegetables grown on their land and fish and sea vegetables from the nearby ocean. I believe this was in line with nature's balance.

THERE IS NO LIVING ENERGY IN CROPS GROWN WITH AGRICULTURAL CHEMICALS

Everything in the natural world is connected. Everything influences everything else, while maintaining a delicate balance. Even those things we feel are "unnecessary" are actually necessary in the natural world.

When cultivating agricultural crops, agricultural chemicals are often used to prevent damage to the crops by harmful insects. However, "harmful insect" is a term made up by humans. In the natural world, there is no such thing as an insect that causes harm.

Humans dislike it when insects get on their agricultural crops, but the truth is, whether harmful or helpful, insects add a certain nutrient to crops when they land on them. That nutrient is chitin-chitosan.

Chitin-chitosan is found in the shells of crab and shrimp, but the hard shell covering insects' bodies is also formed from chitin-chitosan. When insects land on plant leaves of crops, enzymes such as chitonase and chitinase get secreted from the leaves. These enzymes allow the plants to absorb tiny amounts of chitin, about a nanogram or so, from the insect's body, hands and feet, and use that as their own nutrient.

In this way, nutrients that plants absorb from insects contribute to the life of animals that eat those plants.

However, this chain of nutrition is severed by agricultural chemicals. Instead of the insects' chitin-chitosan, the plants and vegetables absorb the agricultural chemicals used to repel insects, in the end causing great harm to humans who eat these plants.

Moreover, agricultural chemicals rob the life of living things in the soil. These living things are the source of energy for agricultural crops. Farmlands periodically sprayed with agricultural chemicals do not even have worms or good soil bacteria. Since crops cannot grow on sterile land with no living energy, chemical fertilizers have to be used. Crops can be grown with such chemical fertilizers, but they are deficient in flavor and nutritive value. This is why nutrients found in agricultural crops are decreasing every year.

Another hazard is created by the irrigation of crops. Water for agricultural use is not sterilized with chlorine like regular tap water. But the water is polluted by agricultural chemicals, river pollution and human sewage. Plenty of water is needed to grow crops. Toxins that enter the human body are, to a certain extent, excreted from the body by drinking water. The same can be said of plants. However, because the crop water that is supposed to excrete toxins from plants is polluted itself, it is inevitable that toxins will accumulate in the crops.

The third problem is greenhouse cultivation. The purpose of utilizing the greenhouse is to reduce damage by harmful insects and to control temperature. However, the downside to this—although not well-known—is that sunlight is blocked out by a vinyl covering. Plants cannot move around like animals. For that reason, they are exposed to large amounts of ultraviolet rays. Ultraviolet rays from the sun cause animals and plants to collect free radicals and oxidize. In order for plants to protect themselves against this, they possess a mechanism that enables them to produce large amounts of antioxidant substances.

These antioxidant agents include vitamins such as A, C and E and polyphenols such as flavanoid, isoflavone and catechin, all of which are found in substantial amounts in plants. These antioxidant substances are produced when plants are exposed to ultraviolet rays. In other words, if you shut out sunlight using vinyl, the intensity of ultraviolet rays shining down on the plants gets reduced. As a result, the plants end up producing fewer antioxidant substances such as vitamins and polyphenols.

In the agricultural industry today, the priority is to produce foods that look nice rather than producing ones with nutritional value. Vegetables grown in nature have insect holes in their leaves, or their shapes may be irregular. In truth, they are not really nice-looking vegetables. But, they possess much more living energy.

Since you get your energy from the foods you eat, if the food itself does not contain any living energy, you will never become healthy no matter how much you eat. A person who does not eat food grown in nature cannot expect to have a healthy life in nature. The food you eat everyday sustains your body and the criteria used to choose that food determine your health condition.

The good news is that a growing number of people are starting to use organic fertilizers and organic farming methods. The cost of these products is certainly more than the cost for "normal" goods, but if you ask me, that is the price of a healthy life, and it is much cheaper than getting sick.

Life is sustained only by food with living energy. Crops with living energy can only be produced on land that possesses living energy. If the soil bacteria are healthy, then the vegetables and fruits will also grow in a healthy way. Foods raised in a healthy way will make human intestinal bacteria healthy.

EVERYTHING IS WRITTEN IN OUR "SCRIPTS OF LIFE"

All of us periodically overlook important relationships by focusing on only one thing. For instance, if we look only at each organ of the body individually, we overlook how the organs interact with and affect each other. Or, if we look only at the body, we neglect the vital inseparability of the body, mind and spirit.

When you are experiencing *mental* pressure, your *body* will quickly be dominated by sympathetic nerves. In contrast, when you are feeling truly happy, your body is dominated by parasympathetic nerves. At night while you are sleeping, your body recovers because it shifts predominately to parasympathetic nerves.

A person who is mentally stressed every day and is too busy to eat right will experience a physical imbalance. There is more than one factor leading to any disease. Everything is connected. Mental factors, physical factors, environmental factors… You fall ill when all of these factors come together to form a bad cycle.

Poor diet produces large amounts of free radicals in the body, but so do negative feelings like hatred, resentment and jealousy, which are equally as destructive to health as poor diet. You can stop drinking, stop smoking, and eat a perfect diet, but if your mental diet is one of anger, stress, and fear, you can still make yourself sick. In order to live a healthy life, it is very important to maintain a mentally harmonious and stable condition.

Among people with the same kind of cancer, there are those who fall ill to cancer and lose their lives in a short period of time, and then there are also those whose cancer does not progress nearly as fast. I believe this difference lies in the "host," or the person who is sick—specifically, the physical stamina of the host. The metastasis and recurrence of cancer are due to the weakening immune system of the host.

In my opinion, the ability to fight off cancer (or any other disease) depends upon the number of source enzymes in the host. If the host has a certain level of source enzymes, there is a better chance it can combat the cancer. On the other hand, if source enzymes are depleted, a much more "aggressive" cancer will develop, because illness can more easily spread throughout the weakened body.

Compared with the lifespan of the universe, humans enjoy a very brief existence, even briefer than that of viruses. One human lifetime passes as quickly as the blink of an eye. Even if I live 120 years, I would consider that a short life. There are so many things I would like to do in this lifetime and the things I would like to accomplish all require constant motivation and a high level of energy. Perhaps you feel the same, and that is why you are reading this book. Because our lives are so short, let us live them in health, happiness and vitality. I tell my patients (and anyone else who will listen) they have the choice to stay young, stay healthy, stay positive and develop interests in many different things.

I realize that our lives, including my own, are only a microcosm of the whole picture. I have a soft spot for all of these small but important lives. Do you not think it is wasteful to lose that short and precious life by muddling along in resentment and fear, eating junk, and suffering with ill health and low energy?

There is no need to get sick and suffer during our short lives because the way to live healthily has already been scripted for each of us. First, you need to listen to what your body is trying to tell you. If you cannot hear that voice, then you need to learn it from nature. If you look at nature's laws, you will realize it is telling us humans exactly what we need right now. If you are humble enough to accept nature's law and entrust yourself to your life script, those miraculous source enzymes will support you for a long, full and happy life.

LOVE ACTIVATES YOUR MIRACLE ENZYME

"Man cannot live by bread alone" is a biblical teaching, but I learned from many patients that it is also one of nature's laws.

There have been cases of very sick people miraculously recovering from illnesses after setting their minds on some goal. There have been cases worldwide in which people suffering from an illness develop, by some incident or other, feelings of gratitude, and once they start having those feelings, they begin to recover.

All humans have infinite potential, but that potential is often hidden. When there is an opening for that potential to be realized, enzymes in the body get activated, creating energy and even bringing people back from near death. On the other hand, no matter how healthy your body is, if you live a life of loneliness, always focusing on the negative and feeling sorry for yourself, your body's enzymes will steadily lose their strength.

I do not think curing cancer through love is an impossibility. If a person truly believes that he or she will be cured and experiences true love from the depths of his or her heart, I believe that person will be able to overcome the disease. If you strongly wish from the bottom of your heart that you want to live, no matter what, to see your beloved children or grandchildren grow up, then chances are you will live to see that happen. Depending on the strength of your will, you can open doors to seemingly impossible possibilities.

In order to cure an illness, the doctor cannot merely cut out the "diseased parts" of the patient's body or just give him or her medicine. Curing means motivating the person so that he or she can feel genuine happiness. A truly great doctor is one who can skillfully provide that kind of motivation. My personal goal is to become that kind of a doctor.

So what would be a strong motivation for such patients? I believe there is no greater motivating factor than love.

We all know there are many forms of love — between a man and a woman, between a parent and child, between companions and friends, between us and people in need — but whatever the form, I believe motivation, wellness and happiness are all born from love. In order to become healthy, it is absolutely necessary to feel love for someone. Few people can be happy alone. A happy life is full of love, and the stages of love evolve from receiving love, building love with others, and giving love.

When a person is truly happy, blood tests will reveal a very active immune system. Since source enzymes heighten your body's immune functions, a person who is feeling happy most likely will have plenty of source enzymes.

Moreover, when you are feeling happy, the parasympathetic nerves of the nervous system take over, thus decreasing your stress level. When your stress level decreases, fewer free radicals are produced, and the intestinal floral balance starts leaning in favor of good bacteria. When your intestinal environment improves, that condition gets transmitted via your parasympathetic nerves to the hypothalamus in the brain, whereupon your cerebrum receives this information and gives you even greater feelings of pleasure.

Feeling of happiness ➜ parasympathetic nerves take over ➜ reduction of stress ➜ improvement of intestinal balance ➜ message via parasympathetic nerves ➜ transmission to hypothalamus ➜ greater feeling of happiness.

Parts of the human body —whether the immune system, endocrine system, or nervous system — do not function alone. They all influence each other. If one good cycle begins, the whole body shifts at once in a positive direction.

When you begin a cycle of happiness, enzymes are produced in large amounts. These enzymes in turn positively stimulate cells throughout the body. Thus, enzymes, which are produced by this cycle of happiness, are actually the ones behind the scenes to activate the self-healing powers of a person who feels happiness through love.

I am sure you will realize that love is a very important heading written in our "life scripts."

Afterword

The Enzyme Factor: From Entropy to Syntropy

I turned 72 in March of 2007, and when I see my classmates from time to time, I can tell what kind of life each of them has lived since we first met. Some look like typical old men, while others look very young. The difference lies in various factors, such as their diet history, lifestyle habits, the water they drink, their sleep patterns, and their living environment and motivation. An older person's body never lies. The body truly reflects the life that has been lived.

Some people say that from the moment we are born, all living things head along the same path towards death. This is true. After all, in keeping with the laws of nature, our lives will one day surely end.

However, the speed at which one walks down that path can vary greatly. People who experience high levels of physical and mental stress may finish their journey in only 40 years, but others can stroll down life's path, taking 100 or so years to reach the end. They can accomplish this by caring for their bodies and minds, and enjoying the scenery along the road with a partner or friends.

The road we choose is determined by our own free will. But since the end result is the same, would it not be better to create and enjoy a long, fruitful life?

Take, as an example, a single nail. That nail will one day rust, eventually crumbling and disintegrating. The nail will rust quickly in a place exposed to salt, such as along the seacoast; but if you regularly apply a coat of paint or oil to the nail's head, you may prevent it from rusting for quite some time.

The process by which anyone or anything heads toward destruction or decay is called "entropy." But the speed of entropy changes greatly depending on the environment. The process of reversing the progression of entropy towards repair, regeneration, and revival is called "syntropy."

Since all of us are destined to die, we can say that life flows along the river of entropy. But at the same time, nature provides all of us with the possibility of syntropy as well. A living thing, creating new life from a part of its body, is engaging in syntropy. In animals, for example, the mother's egg and father's sperm unite to create new life. In plants, even if a plant's trunk decays, a new bud will grow from its seed or the tip of a root. Some fish, like salmon, exchange their own lives to create a new life, swimming upstream to spawn and die. These examples represent the moment when entropy changes to syntropy.

Entropy and syntropy coexist in nature's plan.

The human body regenerates every day through metabolism. Even if we get sick, our natural healing powers help us recover. These are all functions of syntropy. However, in order for our body's syntropy to function normally, we must live according to nature's laws. And throughout this book I have promoted good diet and good lifestyle as ways to live according to those laws.

In humans, there is one other unique factor that can convert our body's entropy to syntropy, and that is our mental strength. I have stressed the importance of motivation and happiness and their role in helping us live healthy lives because I want to emphasize the mind's power and influence on the physical body.

At present, specialized medicine does not truly pay heed to mental factors such as motivation, although motivation greatly influences the body, and it is indispensable for anyone seeking to live an energetic and healthy life.

People who are always in the public eye, such as actors, actresses, politicians and businessmen, often glow with youthful exuberance. Their awareness that they are the center of attention stirs up their motivation. On the other hand, we often hear about how a person—who until recently had been working very hard—suddenly ages or becomes sick the moment he or she retires, no doubt because of a loss of motivation. Men and women who live solely for their jobs and lack outside interests will not know what to do with themselves after they retire. A more balanced person will be more likely to make a healthy transition to his post-retirement life.

If, after reading this book, you start to follow my advice to avoid eating oxidized foods and dairy products, to drink good water, and to focus on feelings of gratitude and happiness every day, your body will begin to shift from a state of entropy to syntropy.

The important thing is to act immediately to maintain the momentum of your motivation. No matter how seriously you *think* you will eat better foods, drink good water, or stop drinking and smoking, if these thoughts are not accompanied by action, you will just end up with feelings of guilt and unfulfilled determination, negative emotions that certainly will not help your health.

Many maladies known as "adult illnesses" in the past are now being called "lifestyle-related illnesses." However, whenever I get the opportunity, I tell people that these are really illnesses stemming from either ignorance or a lack of self-control. These are harsh words, I know, for those who are already ill. And, since many of those people fell ill because they did not acquire the right knowledge, the greatest fault may lie with physicians or the patterns of our society.

Still, I call these illnesses stemming from a lack of self-control because I would like you to clearly understand that if you can control yourself, there are many illnesses you can prevent.

Physicians and societal patterns may be responsible for the lack of correct knowledge on these issues, because physicians are themselves often among the people who most frequently fall ill. Many doctors I know have cancer and diabetes. In fact, several decades ago, I read that the average life expectancy for American doctors was 58 years. In other words, even doctors who are supposedly "disease specialists" lack essential knowledge about food and health.

Although this book was written based on the wealth of clinical cases I have studied, you cannot become healthy by simply reading what I have to say. What will make you healthy is your own daily adherence to the right kinds of activities. The development of good habits, however modest at the beginning, will eventually have a significant impact on your health. And it is *never* too late to start something good.

Although there are differences depending on the area of the body, most of your body's cells usually get replaced every 120 days. Thus, for those of you willing to try the Enzyme Factor Diet and Lifestyle, I advise you first to pursue this for at least four months. If you can convert your body's flow of entropy to syntropy and maintain the syntropy, your body will dramatically change even within four months.

Eat a good diet, master a good lifestyle, drink good water, get plenty of rest, exercise moderately and pursue interests that motivate you, and your body will undoubtedly respond in a positive way. No matter how unhealthy your body may be now, it is continually making an effort to stay healthy. Speaking as a physician, nothing could satisfy me more than if you were to put my suggestions into practice after reading this book and experience a dramatic, positive change to your health.

Dr. Shinya's 7 Golden Keys for Good Health

USE THESE KEYS TO PRESERVE YOUR BODY'S "MIRACLE ENZYME" AND ENJOY A LONG AND HEALTHY LIFE.

1. A GOOD DIET

1. **85–90% Plant-based foods:**

    a. 50% whole grains, brown rice, whole wheat pasta, barley, cereals, whole grain bread & beans including soybeans, kidney beans, garbanzo beans, lentils, pinto beans, pigeon peas, black, white & pink beans

    b. 30% green and yellow vegetables and root vegetables, including potatoes, carrots, yams and beets, and sea vegetables

    c. 5–10% fruits, seeds & nuts

2. **10–15% Animal-based proteins (no more than 3 to 4 oz per day):**

    a. Fish any type but preferably small fish as the larger fish contain mercury

    b. Poultry: chicken, turkey, duck – small amounts only

    c. Beef, lamb, veal pork – should be limited or avoided

    d. Eggs

    e. Soymilk, soy cheese, rice milk, almond milk.

    ### *Foods to add to your diet:*

    1. Herbal teas

    2. Seaweed tablets (kelp)

3. Brewers yeast (good source of B complex vitamins and minerals)

4. Bee pollen and propolis

5. Enzyme supplements

6. Multivitamin & mineral supplement

Foods & substances to avoid or limit in your diet:

1. Dairy products such as cow's milk, cheese, yogurt, other milk products

2. Japanese green tea, Chinese tea, English tea (limit to 1–2 cups per day)

3. Coffee

4. Sweets and sugar

5. Nicotine

6. Alcohol

7. Chocolate

8. Fat and oils

9. Regular table salt (Use sea salt with trace minerals.)

Additional Dietary Recommendations:

1. Stop eating and drinking 4–5 hours before bedtime.

2. Chew every mouthful 30–50 times.

3. Do not eat between meals except for whole fruit (If hunger keeps you awake a piece of whole fruit may be eaten one hour before bedtime as it digests quickly.)

4. Eat fruits and drink juices 30-60 minutes before meals.

5. Eat whole, unrefined grains and cereals.

6. Eat more food raw or lightly steamed. Heating food over 118 degrees will kill enzymes.

7. Do not eat oxidized foods. (Fruit, which has turned brown, has begun to oxidize.)

8. Eat fermented foods.

9. Be disciplined with the food you eat. Remember you are what you eat.

2. Good Water

Water is essential for your health. Drink water with strong reduction power that has not been polluted with chemical substances. Drinking "good water" such as mineral water or hard water, which has much calcium and magnesium, keeps your body at an optimal alkaline pH.

- Adults should drink at least 6–10 cups of water every day.

- Drink 1–3 cups of water after waking up in the morning.

- Drink 2–3 cups of water about one hour before each meal.

3. Regular Elimination

- Start a daily habit to remove intestinal pollutants and to clean out your system regularly.

- Do not take laxatives.

- If the bowel is sluggish or to detoxify the liver, consider using a coffee enema. The coffee enema is better for colon detox and for full body detox because it does not release free radicals into the blood stream, as do some dietary detox methods.

4. MODERATE EXERCISE

- Exercise appropriate for your age and physical condition is necessary for good health but excessive exercise can release free radicals and harm your body.

- Some good forms of exercise are walking (2.5 miles), swimming, tennis, bicycling, golf, muscle strengthening, yoga, martial arts and aerobics.

5. ADEQUATE REST

- Go to bed at the same time every night and get 6 to 8 hours of uninterrupted sleep.

- Do not eat or drink 4 or 5 hours before bedtime, If you are hungry or thirsty a small piece of fruit may be eaten one hour before retiring as it will digest quickly.

- Take a short nap of about 30 minutes after lunch.

6. BREATHING AND MEDITATION

- Practice meditation.

- Practice positive thinking.

- Do deep abdominal breathing 4 or 5 times per hour. The exhale should be twice as long as the inhale. This is very important as deep breaths help to rid the body of toxins and free radicals.

- Wear loose clothing that does not restrict your breath.

- Listen to your own body and be good to yourself.

7. Joy and Love

- Joy and love will boost your body's enzyme factor sometimes in miraculous ways.
- Take time every day for an attitude of appreciation.
- Laugh.
- Sing.
- Dance.
- Live passionately and engage your life, your work, and the ones you love with your full heart.

Recommended Dietary Habits

CHEW YOUR FOOD WELL.

Chew each bite of food 30 to 70 times. Such chewing releases an active secretion of saliva, an enzyme that binds well with gastric juice and bile and aids in the digestion process. Careful chewing increases blood glucose levels which suppress the appetite and curb overeating. It also assists in efficiently absorbing even small amounts of food.

EAT WHOLE GRAINS ORGANICALLY GROWN IF POSSIBLE.

Brown rice, whole grains and beans are very good and fermented foods are great foods. Eat a handful of beans every day. The beans contain more protein than meat and lots of elements including vitamins and minerals and selenium.

EAT ONLY THE MEAT OF ANIMALS WITH A BODY TEMPERATURE LOWER THAN OUR OWN.

It is not good to eat high body temperature animals like beef and chicken because the animal fat will solidify in the human bloodstream. It is much better to eat low body temperature animals like fish because fish oil liquifies in our body and even flushes out the arteries instead of clogging them.

AVOID EATING OR DRINKING PRIOR TO RETIRING FOR THE NIGHT.

It is important to finish eating and drinking 4–5 hours before retiring at night. When the stomach is empty there is a high level of a strong acid that kills Helicobacter pylori bacterium as well as other bad bacteria, creating a balanced intestinal environment that is conducive to self-healing, resistance and immunity. Limiting liquid and food before bedtime also helps prevent acid reflux problems and sleep apnea.

Drink 8–10 glasses of good water per day.

It is important to develop and maintain a good drinking rhythm and timing. Drink two to three cups of water after rising in the morning and two to three cups of water thirty minutes to one hour before each meal. It is important that you drink before the meal rather than with or after the meal, as you don't want to dilute the digestive enzymes. If you must have liquid with your meal, sip only about ½ cup. Good water is water free of substances hazardous to the human body which includes chlorine. Good water has small water clusters and contains an appropriate balance of minerals such as calcium, magnesium, sodium, potassium and iron. The pH index should be above 7.5 or slightly alkali. The water should not have oxidized calcium in high amounts. In short, good water should be capable of eliminating free radicals through anti-oxidation.

Eat quality carbohydrates.

Carbohydrates are easy to digest and absorb as an immediate source of energy. Quality carbohydrates contain dietary fibers, vitamins and minerals, all elements that contribute to efficient cell metabolism, blood flow and elimination of wastes. Carbohydrates of premium quality, when digested and absorbed for energy, produce water and carbon dioxide. They do not produce toxins or waste like that of metabolized proteins or fat. Since carbohydrate metabolism does not dirty the blood with wastes and does not require much energy expenditure to be digested and absorbed, it is an ideal source of energy for activity tolerance and endurance.

Some Sources of high quality carbohydrates:

- Unrefined or brown rice
- Unrefined barley
- Buckwheat
- Millet
- Corn
- Amaranth
- Quinoa
- Whole grain bread
- Dark ground Japanese buckwheat made from unrefined grains

SELECT YOUR DIETARY FAT CAREFULLY.

Fat is categorized by its source – plant or animal.

Plant oils include:

- olive
- soybean
- corn
- sesame
- rapeseed
- saffron
- rice-bran oils

Animal fats include:

- butter
- lard
- fat from meat
- fish oil

Fat is further categorized as containing saturated or unsaturated fatty acids. Saturated fatty acids such as stearic acid and palmitic acid are abundant in animal fat. Unsaturated fatty acids are found in plant oils in the form of linoleic, linolen, aleic and alachidon acids. Linoleic and alachidon acids are called essential fatty acids or vitamin F, which cannot be produced by the body and therefore must be obtained from food. Animal fat promotes the accumulation of wastes, leading to arteriosclerosis, hypertension and obesity. Natural foods such as brown rice, sesame seeds, corn and soybean contain about 30% fat and are a much better source of required fat than that of refined oil because their metabolism does not burden the pancreas and liver. Additionally, plant oils flush out wastes such as bad cholesterol and prevent arteriosclerosis by keeping cells and blood vessels flexible. Vegetable oils sold as salad oils are chemically treated and are not recommended.

EAT FISH OIL.

Fish Oil is good for your brain. High blood levels of DHA found in fish oil has been linked to mathematical and other mental abilities. Although the effects of DHA on the cerebral/nervous system are not specifically understood, it is postulated that DHA lessens the risk of developing dementia or Alzheimer's disease. Some studies show that omega 3 lowers blood triglycerides, reducing the incidence of blood clots.

DECREASE YOUR DEPENDENCE ON DRUGS BY MODIFYING YOUR DIET AND GETTING EXERCISE WHEN POSSIBLE.

Dependence on drugs, even prescription drugs, can be harmful to health because they tax the liver and kidneys. Many chronic conditions such as arthritis, gout, diabetes and osteoporosis can be managed with diet and exercise.

EAT HIGH FIBER FOODS FOR PROPER ELIMINATION
AND TO PREVENT AGE-RELATED DISEASES.

All kinds of dietary fibers exist in various foods. They are abundant in plant-based foods such as vegetables and sea vegetables, fruits, legumes, unrefined grains, cereals and fungi. Dried sea vegetables contain 50–60% dietary fiber by weight. Dietary fiber intake in the form of granules, capsules or liquids is not advisable. These supplements can interfere with the absorption of other nutrients, resulting in disease.

MICRONUTRIENTS HAVE MIRACLE POWER.

Micronutrients include vitamins, minerals, and amino acids. The term "micro" refers to the smaller quantity required as compared with the indispensable "macro" requirements of carbohydrate, protein, fat and dietary fiber. Micronutrients are critical to maintaining health, mental and emotional balance, and preventing disease. Certain amounts of these nutrients are required by the body; these amounts are called the Recommended Daily Allowance. The RDA represents the minimum amount needed to prevent disease. The requirement however differs on an individual basis, depending on the person's diet and lifestyle. Even if one eats the same type and amount of food with the same number of calories each day, the amount of nutrients absorbed and excreted differs dependent on the body's physical, mental or emotional state on that day. A diet of healthy, natural foods in proper proportions does not necessarily guarantee an adequate intake of vitamins, minerals or amino acids.

TAKE SUPPLEMENTS IN MODERATION.

It is important to eat natural foods that are well balanced and synchronized with one's individual biorhythm. Several studies have demonstrated that micro-nutrient supplementation can minimize age-related diseases and improve the cure rates for cancers, heart disease and chronic diseases. The teamwork of all the nutrients is what maintains our health. Taking two or three nutrients with some vitamins and minerals while excluding or minimizing others will make it impossible to maintain a top-notch health status or prevent diseases and the aging process. Consumption of a high dose of a particular vitamin or mineral from among the essential nutrients may be effective for some people but unhealthy for others.

Fat soluble vitamins such as A,D,E and K are stored in the liver and body fat and therefore it is not necessary to supplement these everyday. Water-soluble vitamins, which are vitamin B complexes and vitamin C are soluble in body fluids and excreted in the urine; therefore, a daily intake of these is important, though only small amounts are needed,. *(There is some research that indicates too many supplements can have a negative effect on our immune system, increase free radicals and prompt changes in the fat found in the liver, heart and kidneys.While I recommend supplementation of micro-nutrients, these findings should not be discounted, and I suggest moderation, self- awareness and caution.)*

VITAMINS AND MINERALS WORK TOGETHER

Vitamins are organic, minerals are inorganic. These essential nutrients complement each other in their roles. For example, vitamin D facilitates the absorption of calcium. Vitamin C works to absorb iron; iron expedites the metabolism of the vitamin B groups; copper stimulates the activation of vitamin C and magnesium is necessary to metabolize vitamin C. Integrated functioning of the micronutrients is extensive and yet our current knowledge of these processes is limited.

Minerals strengthen your enzyme factor.

Minerals are required to maintain health. They include:

- calcium
- magnesium
- phosporus
- potassium
- sulfur
- copper
- zinc
- iron
- bromine
- selenium
- iodine
- molybdenum

Minerals play as important a role as that of vitamins in preventing diseases, hypertension, osteoporosis and cancer. Minerals work synergistically with vitamins and enzymes as well as antioxidants in eliminating free radicals. Large quantities of minerals on a daily basis are usually not indicated but deficiencies can create serious health problems. Minerals strengthen immunity and healing and support your own body's enzyme factor.

While vitamins are found in live foods such as plants and animals, minerals are found in the soil, water and the sea (as organic or inorganic salts). The mineral content of foods depends on where the foods are grown as well as the quality of the soil in which they are grown. The minerals in soil can be changed or destroyed by acidic rain or chemical fertilizers. Minerals from vegetables, grains and cereals are easily lost and the refinement process of grains destroys most of the minerals. This makes it difficult to obtain a balanced level of the required minerals from our daily intake of food. Latent deficiencies of minerals manifest as loss of vitality, attention deficit, irritability, overweight and other unhealthy states.

Minerals are water-soluble and are passed through urine and perspiration. The body's consumption of minerals can vary from day to day, depending on our mental and physical activities, stress, exercises, menstruation, pregnancy or chronological age. With certain medications, mineral deficiencies can rapidly develop. Diuretics, oral contraceptives, laxatives, alcohol and smoking accelerate the excretion or destruction of calcium, iron, magnesium, zinc and potassium.

HYPERACTIVITY IN CHILDREN MIGHT REALLY BE A CALCIUM DEFICIENCY.

Studies in recent years show an increase in children with short attention spans who are prone to angry outbursts. Food and nutrition can have a significant impact on a child's behavior and social adaptability. There is a growing tendency for children at home and at school to consume increased amounts of processed foods. Not only do these foods contain several additives, but processed foods tend to make the body acidic. Animal protein and refined sugar are also consumed in increased amounts while vegetables are often avoided. Animal protein and sugar demand increased calcium and magnesium leading to calcium deficiency. Calcium deficiency irritates the nervous system, contributing to nervousness and irritability

EXCESS INTAKE OF CALCIUM AFTER MIDDLE AGE IS HARMFUL.

Calcium prevents cancers, resists stress, reduces fatigue, lowers cholesterol and prevents osteoporosis, but a calcium intake in excess of the daily requirement to correct a deficiency is harmful. I've already described why dairy is an unacceptable way to increase calcium intake. One treatment is a supplement of active vitamin D and calcium. Vitamin D facilitates the absorption of calcium from the small intestine and stimulates bone formation. Excess calcium can cause constipation, nausea, loss of appetite and abdominal distention. If taken without food, calcium thins gastric acid promoting an imbalance of intestinal bacteria and poor absorption of iron, zinc and magnesium. If you need to supplement calcium, the recommended daily intake is 800 to 1500 mg, taken in 3 doses of 250 to 500 mg with meals. The balance of calcium with other minerals and vitamins is a critical component of good health.

MAGNESIUM ACTIVATES HUNDREDS OF DIFFERENT ENZYMES AND IS A TREATMENT FOR MIGRAINE AND DIABETES.

Magnesium is an important mineral and large amounts are required to maintain good health. Its deficiency is manifested by irritability, anxiety, depression, dizziness, weakened muscles, muscle spasm, heart disease and hypertension. A recent study in Germany indicated that patients who had a heart attack had low magnesium levels. Research in the U.S. reported that 65% of migraine patients tested experienced complete relief after taking 100-200 mg of magnesium. Low magnesium impairs glucose tolerance. Hence diabetes management is improved when appropriate magnesium levels are maintained.

A BALANCE OF SODIUM AND POTASSIUM IS A PREREQUISITE FOR LIFE.

Sodium is well known as salt. This mineral is responsible for maintaining fluid balance both inside and outside of body cells. Sodium maintains the correct pH (acid/alkaline level) in the blood and is an indispensable element for the proper functioning of gastric acid, muscles and nerves. Sodium is abundant in life, but deficiency can easily evolve from a large intake of laxatives and extended periods of diarrhea or vigorous sports or activities, particularly in hot weather. A balance of sodium and potassium is a prerequisite of life. The balance between sodium and potassium effects fluid shifts inside and outside of cells. Sodium is normally found outside the cell. When potassium in the fluid inside the cell is low, sodium, with fluid, rushes into the cell, causing it to swell. The increase in cell size places pressure on the veins, narrowing the vessel's diameter and is a factor in hypertension. The ratio of sodium to potassium ideally is one to one, but many processed foods contain sodium, and sodium can be consumed in excess without our awareness.

With sufficient intake of vegetables and their juice, potassium is supplied to restore balance with the amount of sodium present.

SMALL QUANTITIES OF TRACE MINERALS WORK SYNERGISTICALLY WITH VITAMINS, MINERALS AND ENZYMES.

Trace minerals are critical to support our life. The amounts required are small but their importance cannot be ignored. They support balance and harmony in our body functions. After absorption through the intestines, these minerals are ferried through the circulatory system to cells entering through the cell's membrane. The most important fact to remember is that the intake of these minerals must be properly balanced. One or two of these trace minerals in large amounts will result in the loss of other minerals and malabsorption. Thus, it is best to get these trace minerals from our food rather than supplements. Sea salt and sea vegetables are good sources.

- **Boran**: important for the absorption of calcium and maintenance of teeth and bones.

- **Copper**: generates bone, hemoglobin and red blood cells; generates elastin and collagen lowers cholesterol levels and increases HDL cholesterol. (Excess copper has been found in patients with malignant tumors especially of the digestive tract, lung and breast so their may be a link with the development of cancer.)

- **Zinc**: plays a role in the production of insulin; metabolizes carbohydrates, creates protein and absorbs vitamins, particularly B, from the digestive tract; maintains prostate function and supports male reproductive health

- **Iron**: core component of hemoglobin and plays a role in the function of enzymes, the B complex vitamins and resistance to disease

- **Selenium**: prevents free radical production when combined with Vitamin E. This is a wonder mineral found in soil deposits. (The soil in Cheyenne, Wyoming contains high amounts of selenium compared to that of Muncee, Indiana. The death rate from cancer in Cheyenne is 25% lower than that in Muncee.) Studies indicate that with insufficient selenium there is an increased incidence of prostate, pancreatic, breasst, ovarian, skin, lung, rectal-colon and bladder cancers as well as leukemia.

- **Chromium**: facilitates the metabolism of carbohydrates and protein; facilitates glucose metabolism maintaining a blood glucose level that does not demand excessive insulin utilization preventing hypoglycemia and diabetes.

- **Manganese**: metabolizes protein and fat and creates hormones.

- **Molybdenum**: promotes healthy teeth and mouth.

- **Iodine**: critical for the normal functioning of the thyroid gland and the prevention of goiter development.

Healing Foods

Sea Vegetables are a great source of dietary fiber. Insoluble dietary fibers that are indigestible absorb water in the intestines, adding bulk to the intestinal walls and accelerating peristaltic movement. In this way they prevent the accumulation of toxins in the colon.

Nori is the Japanese name for various edible seaweed species of the red alga Porphyra including most notably P. yezoensis and P. tenera. The term nori is also commonly used to refer to the food products created from these so-called "sea vegetables"

Kanten a sea plant rich in vitamins, minerals & trace minerals including iodine, calcium & iron.

Hijiki (Hizikia fusiformes) is a sea vegetable growing wild around the coasts of Japan. Hijiki is known to be rich in dietary fibre and essential minerals. Japanese women believe Hijiki will make the hair thick and healthy.

Aonori is rich in iron, potassium and Vitamin C, It contributes to collagen and elastin production in skin and is known for its anti-aging properties.

Wakame is a sea vegetable found in the waters of Japan. A compound in wakame helps burn fat.

Kima is an edible mushroom from Syria valued as an immune booster.

Maitake is the Japanese name for the edible fungus. Maitake has been used traditionally both as a food and for medicinal purposes. Extracts of maitake mushroom boost the immune system and are hypothesized to have anti-tumor effects.

Kikurage is a fungus that when sliced and cooked with just about anything (great in stir fries and soups) imparts a crunchy texture and mild flavor that goes well with all. They're also renowned for their health-giving properties

Enzyme Factor 1 (Enzyme-x-bio) is a fermented fruit and vegetable enzyme supplement. Beneficial microorganisms have been bought up carefully for dozens of years in koji (Aspergillus oryzea), bacillus natto and other plant yeasts. Fresh seasonal fruits and vegetables are added to this microbial culture and go through the fermentation process. Enzyme Factor-1 contains the optimal balance of various plant enzymes, microbe enzymes and useful microbes to enhance the digestion, promote detoxification, and support cell restoration. Moreover, these microbes are kept in the best condition where they are hibernating and ready to become active when taken into the body.

Siegen enhances the immune system, and improves intestinal bacteria floras and functions. Siegen is composed of excipient extracts from soymilk fermented by a combination of sixteen kinds of lactobacillus and yeasts. When the Lactobacillus Fermented Extracts are concentrated, solubilized microbial constituents are added. Microbial constituents such as peptidoglycans and MDP (muramyl dipeptide) are substances that have attracted attention because of their action on the immune system. Ingredients include: Lactobacillus Fermented Extracts, Cell walls, γ-Cyclodextrin, Dextrin, fructooligosaccharide, Citric acid, Lemon oil, Amino acids(Glutamic acid, Aspartic acid, lysine, Alanine, Glycine, Proline, Histidine, Threonine, Arginine etc). Vitamins(vitamin B1, B2, B6). Mineral(Potassium, Calsium, Magnesium, Phosphorus), Butyric acid, Acetic acid, Lactic acid, Propionic acid, Isoflavones, Saponins.

OrzaeBio is an anti-aging functional food which has antioxidant properties, can improve brain function, and strengthen the immune system. OrzaeBio is fermented ancient rice (FAR). FAR was developed as a collaborated effort between Hirosaki University (Japan) and Origin Biomedical Laboratory (Japan). The main active ingredients are hemicilluloses, oligosaccharide (oryzlose), gamma-amino betyric acid (baga) and anthocyanim. Ingredients include fermented ancient rice bran, maltose and crystal cellulose.

Chaga (Chaga-inonotus obliquus) is a woody mushroom that grows on birch trees. It is an antiviral, anti-tumor remedy sometimes used as a natural medicine for breast, uterine and other cancers as well as diabetes. It is believed to improve immunity and longevity by increasing the vital life force and strengthening the immune system, as an immune amphoteric, also sometimes used for reducing blood pressure and slowing down heart rate.

While Chaga can and does occur on white birch trees in parts of Canada, Japan, and northern Scandinavia, the highest quality specimens are found in Russia from the black birch trees of Siberia. Chaga has a black, scarred outer surface that looks like burnt charcoal with a light brown interior. It is most often consumed in a hot tea mixture, Chaga has been used as a traditional medicine in Russia and Eastern Europe for at least fifteen hundred years for a variety of diseases, including stomach pain, ulcers, asthma, bronchitis, liver problems, and even cancer.

Kotosugi (Taxaceae) is an evergreen tree mainly distributed in the Yunnan Province of China. Koto means red bean and sugi means sugar from cedar. The wood has been used as a traditional Chinese Royal medicine for over 2000 years. In 1971 the anti-cancer ability of the Kotosugi tree was investigated and resulted in isolating the compound taxol. Today, taxol has been synthesized and has been shown to be an effective anti-cancer treatment. Taxol is a tubulin-binder, which inhibits cell division. As a powerful cancer drug Taxol can have unwanted side effects.

When taken as a tea red bean ceda (kotosugi) is empirically known to be non-toxic to the human body.

Kangen Water is alkaline rich water (ph 8-9), and is considered the very best drinking water because of its incomparable powers of hydration, detoxification, and anti-oxidation.

For more information visit www.enzymefactor.com

Index